Developing Early Verbal Skills Through Music

of related interest

Music, Language and Autism
Exceptional Strategies for Exceptional Minds
Adam Ockelford
Foreword by Francesca Happé
ISBN 978 1 84905 197 2
eISBN 978 0 85700 428 4

Music for Special Kids
Musical Activities, Songs, Instruments and Resources
Pamela Ott
ISBN 978 1 84905 858 2
eISBN 978 0 85700 426 0

Early Childhood Music Therapy and Autism Spectrum Disorders
Developing Potential in Young Children and Their Families
Edited by Petra Kern and Marcia Humpal
ISBN 978 1 78592 775 1
eISBN 978 1 78450 688 9

**Developmental Speech-Language Training through Music
for Children with Autism Spectrum Disorders**
Theory and Clinical Application
Hayoung A. Lim
ISBN 978 1 84905 849 0
eISBN 978 0 85700 415 4

Speak, Move, Play and Learn with Children on the Autism Spectrum
Activities to Boost Communication Skills, Sensory Integration and Coordination Using
Simple Ideas from Speech and Language Pathology and Occupational Therapy
Lois Jean Brady, America X Gonzalez, Maciej Zawadzki and Corinda Presley
ISBN 978 1 84905 872 8
eISBN 978 0 85700 531 1

DEVELOPING EARLY VERBAL SKILLS THROUGH MUSIC

Using Rhythm, Movement and Song with Children and Young People with Additional or Complex Needs

TRACY JEFFERY

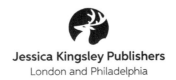

Jessica Kingsley Publishers
London and Philadelphia

First published in Great Britain in 2023 by Jessica Kingsley Publishers
An imprint of John Murray Press

I

A CIP catalogue record for this title is available from the
British Library and the Library of Congress

ISBN 978 1 78775 883 4
eISBN 978 1 78775 884 1

Printed and bound by CPI Group (UK) Ltd, Croydon, CR0 4YY

Jessica Kingsley Publishers
Carmelite House
50 Victoria Embankment
London EC4Y 0DZ

www.jkp.com

John Murray Press
Part of Hodder & Stoughton Limited
An Hachette UK Company

This book is dedicated to Damaris, Graham, and Mum and Dad, with all my love and to all the children and young people I have taught and learned from since my first cautious step into a music session 20 years ago, especially those who sang but did not speak.

Acknowledgements

Very, very special thanks to my husband, Graham Viktor Perkins, who patiently and perfectly crafted the technical figures for this book from the scraps I gave him, mastered endless forms of new technology to fix the videos, and spotted their typos and erroneous en-dashes. Thank you for making me raise my game, and for keeping me going when the whole project felt just too big – as it often did. This book would not have happened without you.

Assembling this book took two years, from conception to first draft, but its roots go back decades. I owe thanks and gratitude to my family who raised me on music, science and debate: especially to my mum, Clair, and my grandparents who filled the house with music and sound of so many genres. And to my dad, who preferred silence, but who helped me get my head around physics at O-level: it was having an oscilloscope in the house that led to me exploring voice through acoustic analysis decades later.

I also owe thanks to my MSc and PhD supervisor, Sandra Whiteside, who taught me to be rigorous in my arguments; and to my wonderful colleagues who have been so generous with their encouragement, wisdom and support: Alison, Craig, Hadiza, Julia and Maria. Special thanks to Julia Lindley-Baker, who heard my request to do some research, made it happen, and opened so many new doors that led me here.

Thank you to everyone who contributed their expertise and insight to the book and online materials: Dr Hadiza Kere Abdulrahman; Craig, Lisa and Annie Bridge; Tracey Gjertsen, chartered physiotherapist: Alexandra Jai and Michael Millman of Rhythm Bliss; and Alison Taylor. Thank you to all who read drafts, and who challenged my words, thinking or perspective: Craig Bridge, Jack Broadbent, Sue Buckley, Alexander Cassidy, Emily Holford, Gillian Howard, Graham Miller, Kerry Miller,

Andrea Porter, Becky Sandford, Alan Trench, Damaris Trench, Emma Wren.

Finally, thank you to Elen, Maudisa and Emma at JKP for all their hard work in moving this book from an idea to reality.

CREDITS

All figures have been created by Tracy Jeffery and Graham Viktor Perkins. Some images have been adapted from images available in research literature: these are credited.

All case studies are based on my teaching and research practice, but names and other identifying features have been changed. Participants of my MSc and PhD gave consent for me to share anonymized speech samples: all speech samples in the online resources are treated to remove names and speech characteristics that could identify them. Permission was given to use direct quotations by participants of my 2021 study of voice in hypermobility spectrum disorders.

Contents

Introduction

THE BIG QUESTIONS

What is the book about? Who is this book written for and what types of learner is it relevant to? What topics does the book cover?

By the end of this chapter, you will know:

- what the book is about and what it hopes to achieve
- who might benefit from developing music skills for speech
- what skills, knowledge and abilities you and the learner need before you get started
- what you will know and be able to do when you have finished the book
- the main content of each chapter.

Shhhh...can you hear that? Something amazing happened in your brain, just then, and it is happening right now as you continue to read. You read that /sh/ as a sound and interpreted it as an instruction to quieten or listen: a consequence of having learned to associate the written symbol with a sound, and the sound with its meaning. Your brain produced an electrical version of the sound's acoustic wave shape, allowing you to hear the simple instruction, even though no mouth uttered it (Moro, 2016). Your brain might also have looked up the instructions for making the /sh/ sound, in readiness for you to raise your tongue forward to your soft palate, and to pass breath from your lungs through the gap at great pressure, generating a complex energy signal composed entirely of air.

Now, not all of us do hear text as we read; but most of us do – 80 per cent, in fact (Vilhauer, 2017); and we might also read words in voices that belong, by rights, to other people. How do we get here – from sound to word and symbol, and back again? And what is the role of music in this learning journey? As adults, we have hundreds of words to describe the sounds we hear and make; words such as chime, buzz, crackle, pop, chorus, blare, chatter, mutter, growl, glide, speak, sing. Each captures a subtle difference in acoustic quality, drawing our attention to tone, timbre, loudness, duration, resonance, harshness or pleasantness. But to the newborn infant, the sonic landscape is just *sound*; undifferentiated, complex layers of ever-changing noise. As babies, we begin to sort and separate the noise into strands as our auditory system matures and our brain learns which noises matter and which we can safely ignore (Lenneberg, 1967). As we become experts in our sonic environment, we learn to match specific sounds to people, events, animals and objects, or to our own movements and emotional states. Over the first few years of life, we pay special attention to the sounds that make up words and to the sounds that communicate something vital to us or about us. Music plays an important role in this early learning: we especially love song – it gets our attention better than speech, helps us decode sounds and meaning, and it entertains us and soothes us. Later, as we refine our skills in moving, playing and singing to music, our musical development can continue to support our language and speech skills; and vice versa.

At least, this is all true for the neurotypical brain: those who are born with intact senses and motor skills, and a certain way of processing sensory information. But what about those who do not progress like this? What about the children whose ears, brains or bodies develop differently or more slowly, resulting in altered perception, processing or movement? For these, is this symbiotic relationship between song, music and speech changed: is it weakened or strengthened? There is mounting evidence that music can improve how the brain processes sound, with benefits to language and speech. The big question is: can music help young people who are in the early stages of verbal learning to understand and produce words more easily or more efficiently than speech alone?

This book attempts to answer these questions, based on the current research evidence. It aims to help you learn *why* music can support early verbal learning, and what adaptations you might make to support musical development in people who have additional or complex needs. The research evidence strongly indicates that if we can support learners to develop their skills in perceiving and making music, then we can use music to support skills that they need for learning to speak. Specifically, I argue that we can use musical activities to:

- support perception of speech sounds and rhythm in speech

- motivate vocal, verbal and social communication
- support the body in producing voice and rhythmic movements
- help verbal learners to reproduce spoken words and short phrases more easily
- prime the brain and body for speaking learned words and phrases.

I do not argue that learning will progress beyond early verbal learning skills because the next step is language. The leap from words to language is big: it takes more time to master and places additional pressure on the cognitive, vocal and verbal systems. Currently, there is less robust evidence that skills from music transfer to language; and no research-based evidence that examines transfer to language in people with complex communicative, sensory or cognitive needs. Smaller steps are more realistic and achievable for those who struggle with language and communication, and these are supported with more substantial evidence.

In this book, I explain why some children and young people have difficulties with skills that are common to music and speech – sound, pulse, rhythm, breathing and voice. I explain how and why musical skills can be used to support speech perception, speech production or both, and I offer examples of activities and adaptations so you can begin to support their musical development, if appropriate. We need to understand potential barriers to musical and verbal development so we know how to adapt our teaching to help them make progress. However, you must decide – with the young person, ideally – whether to use music this way. For example, is it in the young person's interests to use their voice to communicate, to produce sounds more clearly, or to develop skills in prosody? Or would an alternative form of communication, or an adaptation on our part, be more appropriate? As we will see, music can support many skills that can improve a young person's quality of life but they must be your guide.

WHO IS THE BOOK ABOUT?

This book will explore the connections between music and speech in children, teenagers and young adults who are in the early stages of verbal development. I am using the term 'early verbal development' to refer to the types of skills that most young children develop by the age of about two to three years – these include the ability to perceive speech sounds and words in speech; the ability to produce words with rhythm, stress and intonation; and the ability to use words and sounds to communicate meaning.

The specific skills and areas of difficulty that I discuss in this book include:

- perception of speech sounds
- phonological awareness
- perception of rhythm in speech and words
- activating the voice for speech and singing
- controlling the voice when speaking or singing
- controlling the body and breath for speaking and singing
- reproducing the rhythm and melody of words or short phrases
- producing rhythmic movements
- entraining movements to a sound or person.

These areas are underpinned by a range of abilities, including cognitive, physiological, social and emotional skills. The people who may benefit from activities in this book will probably have one or more of the following types of difficulty (for readers who are uncertain what these labels mean, please see Appendix 1 in the online resources for explanations):

- physiological differences that affect independent mobility and movement
- hearing impairment
- sensory processing difficulties – auditory processing differences; hyper- or hyposensitivity; altered proprioception
- neurological differences that affect their voice/speech
- motor or muscle differences that affect their voice/speech
- problems with social synchrony
- difficulties with attending to sound
- difficulties holding information in their auditory-verbal memory.

Each chapter in the book will explain how these differences can affect verbal and musical ability, and how and why specific musical activities can support skills for verbal learning. These types of learning differences and difficulties commonly occur in people who are diagnosed with *attention deficit/hyperactivity disorder* (ADHD), *autism, cerebral palsy, developmental language disorder* (previously, *specific language impairment*), *Down syndrome, dyspraxia*, and *hypermobility spectrum disorders/Ehlers Danlos syndrome* (*HSD/h-EDS*), among others.

WHAT IS THE IDEAL AGE OF THE TARGET GROUP?

The information in this book is relevant to very young neurotypical children who are meeting their developmental milestones, and to children and young adults (up to about 25 years) who have neurological differences, developmental delays or complex needs. The ideas and activities herein may be useful for learners of any age, from birth to old age. However, if we want music skills to support verbal learning, activities may have the greatest effect before the brain matures (early twenties). Our brains are most plastic – that is, they learn and adapt easily – when we are young, and research shows that music is most effective in changing the brain when training begins early. However, some people are born with brains that are less plastic, or that develop in a different way or at a different pace. This means that in practice, we should expect changes to happen, but we must also accept that the effects of these changes could take time to develop or show. A longer learning time may be needed for older children and adults, and in those with more complex physical, sensory or learning needs.

WHAT SKILLS DOES THE LEARNER NEED?

Some information will be of value to learners who are still developing the precursors to language, but to take part in the activities I describe, the child or young adult needs to be ready for verbal learning. For example, they must show an interest in speech and sound, even if they do not use their voice or form words. Some chapters focus on the skills we need to produce voice and speech – the expressive verbal skills. To benefit from these, the young person must be starting to use their voice for self-expression. For example, they might be able to use single words; or to use their voice to sing along with someone. They also need some hearing ability: I do discuss how to adapt activities for hearing impairment, but deaf children and young people may benefit from more specialist resources.

The young person might need to have some independent motor control. A greater degree of independent mobility is needed for rhythm work and singing. For learners who do not yet have volitional motor control, music can benefit social inclusion, perception, enjoyment and wellbeing.

Depending on their age, developmental rate and other needs, some children and young people who are pre-verbal might also be at very early stages of exploring sound. I recommend working with the Sounds of Intent (SOI) framework alongside the ideas in this book: the SOI framework identifies skills in listening, responding and creating music that can support learners with a range of needs and abilities. The framework, and related app and website, provide excellent examples of how to support very early listening and responding skills through music, and provides a clear way of measuring progress in early communicative skills. The framework and related materials can be found at https://soundsofintent.app. The online resources include video examples that give you ideas of how musical learning can progress along this framework, too. If you watch these videos, you can see how music supports early verbal skills, too, for some, and how others use music instead of verbal communication.

Finally, the learner needs to be able to tolerate the sounds you explore together, and to have an interest in music. While music-making can help people with sound sensitivity to tolerate noises, you might need to find out about the learner's preferences and tolerance. The information in Chapter 1 can help you explore this further.

DO I NEED ANY SPECIALIST KNOWLEDGE OR SKILLS?

No, you do not need knowledge of learning needs or disabilities, or of music. I have included case studies to help you understand some types of learning difference and disability, so a fundamental knowledge of – or interest in – disability will be enough to get you started. This book is designed for students, teachers, parents, carers, musicians, therapists and anyone interested in how music can support early verbal skills and speech. Accordingly, many of you will have expertise in at least one area – beyond what I offer here – but I hope that the combinations of topics will give even the specialist something new.

You will not need any specific skills in music-making or music theory. The book focuses on the development of early music skills – the type that most of us learned without even thinking about it. I provide explanations and examples of musical games and activities to enable you to try them out for yourself. If you are a professional musician, you will have a head start – but maybe the discussion of challenges to learning skills will be of specific interest to you.

Probably the most critical skills you need are *observation* and the ability to *communicate feedback*. You will need to be able to observe the responses and movements of the people you work with, and give them feedback in some modality (verbal, touch, visual, technological) on what they need to do to improve. It might be helpful to document the different abilities of the people you work with (e.g. their motor skills, functional communication skills) or gather this information from colleagues, parents and professionals.

WHAT TYPES OF MUSIC ACTIVITIES FEATURE IN THIS BOOK?

The types of activities I describe are based on the teachings of Zoltán Kodály (1882–1967) and Émile Jaques-Dalcroze (1865–1950). Their approaches are developmental: that is, they build skills in stages, starting from where the child currently is, and develop new skills through listening, singing and movement. Furthermore, the Kodály approach is based on observations of how children learn language (Houlahan & Tacka, 2015). The methods work on the principles of 'embodiment' – that is, there is an emphasis on movement skills, and on feeling and noticing what is happening in the body. As we explore in Chapter 1, all sound is based in movement. Speech is linked strongly to movement areas in the brain and through movement, we can learn to hear, feel and make highly complex abstract patterns of music. The approaches of Kodály and Dalcroze, and similar developmental methods such as Suzuki or Orff, are commonly used in the research that explores how music training can support language. These methods are known to cause changes in the brain that improve aspects of language learning.

Kodály approaches use games, songs and movement to teach singing, aural learning and music literacy; these activities can be adapted to suit different physical and cognitive needs; some can even be silent. This was the approach that I used when I began teaching people with complex needs, in combination with basic movement activities based on Dalcroze eurhythmics. These methods allowed my non-verbal, noise-sensitive learners to participate in active learning and enabled me to measure and track their musical progress easily. Using this approach, I began to learn what my students might be capable of. My non-verbal students led singing games and demonstrated learning of pitch through gesture and visual images; most learned to compose and play rhythms based on simplified music notation; and some also learned to play colour-coded melodic instruments.

In the book, I offer example activities to illustrate how you might use a musical activity and how you might adapt teaching to support learning. I do not aim to provide comprehensive examples or guidance on music activities – there are plenty of existing resources available that will do this, and I will signpost these in each chapter. Instead, I aim to illustrate how and why you might use specific activities to support specific verbal or communicative skills. In the online resources, I provide videos, sample programmes and downloadable worksheets to demonstrate how you might embed different skills into a single session, with adaptations to meet individual needs. These worksheets and games are based on those I used when I taught 'music for communication' sessions with young adults. The worksheets can help you get a sense of what level a learner is 'at', alongside musical development milestones. There are several videos (numbered 1-10 in the book) that help explain concepts and demonstrate activities. Please visit https://library.jkp.com/redeem and use the code TDDBQQL to download the accompanying video/music/PDFs.

WHEN I HAVE READ THE BOOK, WHAT WILL I KNOW AND BE ABLE TO DO?

By the end of the book, you will know how and why we can use the building blocks of music to support developing speech in children and young adults; you will know what types of adaptations you can make to support the development of musical ability in learners with additional needs; and you will understand both the potential and the limitations of using music for supporting verbal development in children and young adults with quite complex additional needs.

Ultimately, I hope that as you read this book, you will develop confidence in explaining how and why musical activities might benefit those you work with, in terms of speech and, more broadly, in terms of wellbeing.

CONTENT AND STRUCTURE OF THE BOOK

The book contains an introductory chapter, two main parts (rhythm skills, vocal skills) and a concluding chapter (see below). Within each part, each chapter builds on the previous chapters. We begin with the skills that are foundational to advanced skills. However, each chapter can also be used in isolation, so that you can use the aspects that are of most interest or relevance.

I begin each chapter with the 'big questions' that I address; the learning outcomes, and an overview of 'who' the chapter may be most useful for, in terms of different learning needs and labels. All chapters conclude with a summary, and with recommended reading or resources.

I have aimed to keep references 'light' to help maintain flow when reading. Mostly, I have provided references to support arguments about the potential value (or limitations) of using music to support speech and language; and to signpost you to key sources. I have picked out example sources in the text but the Bibliography includes the full body of reading that I used when writing this book.

Chapter descriptions

Chapter 1: Sound Beginnings. In this chapter, we consider what sound is and how we hear it, and why some people might perceive sound differently from us. We look at the links between sound, music, emotion and language; and at theories that explain why music can be used to develop skills for language. As any learner must make progress in musical learning before changes transfer to the verbal domain, we will review what we know about the ways people with different abilities learn and progress in music.

Chapter 2: Finding the Heartbeat of Music and Speech. This chapter explores the connections between beat entrainment (playing in time to another beat), speech perception and language ability. I use case studies to show why some people with sensory, physical and cognitive differences can have difficulties matching movement to a beat; and suggest ways to adapt activities to help them develop their basic skills in beat timing. This is possibly the most important skill we can develop to assist speech perception, and it can support skills for literacy.

Chapter 3: Rhythmic Connections – Communication, Music and Verbal Language. Chapter 3 begins by examining the role of rhythm in social interaction – these skills are a precursor to communication and are needed for music-making activities. I review the similarities and differences between rhythm in music and rhythm in speech, and introduce the PRISM theory that explains why rhythm can support verbal development. I explain how most children develop skills in rhythm for music and speech, from birth to early childhood; and review studies that show how training in rhythm can improve speech.

Chapter 4: Understanding Rhythm Difficulties in Communication, Speech and Music. This chapter examines the types of difficulties that people can have in perceiving and producing rhythm in speech. First, we consider how social and sensory difficulties impact communication in people on the autism spectrum and those with ADHD. Next, I explain how motor-movement difficulties affect speech and musical rhythms, with a focus on people who stutter, and people with Down syndrome.

Chapter 5: Making Rhythm Work for Social Communication and Speech. This chapter describes practical activities that can be adapted to meet different learning abilities and specific speech-related goals. I provide ideas for adapting rhythm activities to support an individual's musical development alongside their speech skills.

Chapter 6: The Foundations of Voice: Breathing and Posture. In this chapter, I explain why some people find it difficult to control their breath for speech or singing. We focus on the types of breathing problems common in Down syndrome, hypermobility spectrum disorder, autism, ADHD and other sensory and processing disorders. The chapter provides examples of activities from chartered physiotherapist Tracey Gjertsen that can be used to support the breath and body as it is needed for voice; and ideas for using music to support breathing for singing and speech.

Chapter 7: Producing Voice. This chapter explains how we use the body to 'construct' voice and what needs to happen for us to sing a note. It provides a brief overview of the types of voice disorders that you might encounter, and the main developmental, physiological, psychological and cognitive issues that can interfere with efficient phonation.

Chapter 8: Understanding and Supporting Voice Difficulties. In this chapter, I focus on the types of voice difficulties that are common in Down syndrome, hypermobility spectrum disorder, autism, ADHD and other sensory and processing disorders. The chapter provides examples of activities that can be used to support the voice.

Chapter 9: Using Singing and Songs for Speech. In this chapter, we consider why singing may be more effective than speech and review the evidence for this. I give an overview of how we learn to sing, and explain some of the difficulties and barriers that some children and young people face when singing songs. Finally, I offer guidance to help you use singing activities and songs to develop different aspects of speech intelligibility, including articulation, fluency and intonation.

Chapter 10: Making Music Work for Speech and Wellbeing. The final chapter focuses on the practicalities of using music to support language. I revisit the OPERA (Patel, 2011, 2014) and PRISM (Fiveash *et al.*, 2021) hypotheses to identify how we can meet these criteria when making music, and consider how we manage this while also supporting learners' enjoyment of music. I explore how sessions can be adapted to meet multiple learning needs, while ensuring that there is a balance between skill development and enjoyment.

Appendices. These online resources include documents that you might find helpful, including definitions of learning differences and difficulties referred to in the book (Appendix 1); worksheets to help you observe skills in pulse, rhythm and song (Appendix 2); and example programmes of music activities for groups who are at different developmental levels (Appendix 3). In Appendix 4, I analyse a musical game that can be used for a group of learners of mixed ability. I explain which cognitive, social, physical and sensory skills we use when playing it, and show how you could adapt the activity to suit the needs of individuals.

RECOMMENDED READING AND RESOURCES

Moro, A. (2016). *Impossible Languages*. Cambridge, MA: MIT Press.
https://kodaly.org.uk/about-us/kodaly-approach.
https://dalcroze.org.uk.
www.soundsofintent.org.

CHAPTER 1

Sound Beginnings

THE BIG QUESTIONS

Why are sound and music so valuable as therapy, especially for verbal learning? What sorts of things should you consider when using sound and music with children and young people?

By the end of this chapter, you will:

- know the basics of how we perceive sound
- understand why others might respond to sound differently from us
- know a little of music's history as a therapy
- understand why music can support language and speech
- know some of the ways people with developmental differences can succeed in music.

WHO IS THIS FOR?

This chapter is for anyone interested in sound and music and their relation to emotion and communication.

It is especially relevant when working with learners who have sensory or perceptual differences, including those with autism, hearing impairment, developmental differences and physical differences. It is also applicable to very young infants, in general.

Case study: James

James burst through the open door, headphones on, his glasses smeared and awry, beaming and quietly singing. Ignoring me, he headed for the middle of the small music room, where he paused. The room was in disarray following the afternoon's 'music for communication' session that had finished moments ago; it was a shambles of instruments and chairs, but it was empty of people. Muttering quietly, James encircled himself with musical equipment. Four flat, brightly-coloured switches formed an arc at his feet, and to his sides, he angled a Soundbeam: each small, red device emitted a 1.5-metre ultrasonic beam and connected via cables to a midi controller on a trolley to his right. James selected a battered African djembe from the scattered percussion around him and declared, 'Ah, that's it!' Cradling the drum in his right arm, he beat a pattern on its skin with his left hand. As he drummed, he twisted and swayed so that his movements interrupted in turn each invisible beam at different points along their lengths, triggering tuneful notes and arpeggios of orchestral sounds. As his tapping feet conjured a timpani, James became a one-man orchestra: composer, conductor, rhythm section and symphony. For more than ten minutes, James just played, smiling and engrossed, the centre of his own musical universe. Then he put down the drum and left without a word or a glance, returning to his footbath and bubbles in the room next door.

James was a young man with *musicality* – an easy ability to create sonic landscapes that had rhythm, form and harmonious textures. He was one of my first students, and he was hard to connect with, at first. The first time we met, he sat in a corner, headphones on, and sobbed, politely refusing to look at his fellow students or me, but not choosing to leave. Like so many young people, James came with labels – *non-verbal, autism, Down syndrome, hearing-impaired* – a set of words that position us as outsiders and separate us. Music offered a bridge: a language-less means of connection. Although he sat apart from the group in our first weeks, he remained with us. The private sonic world that James experienced through his headphones offered him security, safety, predictability and reassurance: and once he learned that he was allowed to keep them on, he began to take small steps into our world. He might listen silently with us all – headphones shifted – to 'The Flower Duet', or 'The Lark Ascending', smiling at us, his eyes streaming tears, or he would sing his favourite songs, headphones on, feet submerged in an aromatherapy footbath, pausing only to blow bubbles through a wand, and kisses to staff as they worked around him. With headphones on, James could keep one foot in his own world and another in ours. Sometimes, he would remove his headphones and emerge fully into our busy, unpredictable social world. He would choose a song for us all to sing; or sing me an opening line as an invite to duet. Or, from his lone position on the outskirts of the group, he would pick up a drum and lead us in a musical game, playing with exquisite musicality as he controlled dynamics, pace and structure. He would then replace his headphones and retreat, watching, with an ear to us and an ear to the world he chose.

James is not an isolated case: many people will have met someone like him – someone whose world seems to exist in parallel to mine or yours and who we only really meet when we shift *our* perspective or way of communicating. For James and so many others like him who enjoy music, we can use music as our main medium of communication, and we can use it to encourage and foster non-verbal and verbal skills. Music offers learners like James tools to connect and communicate if they choose. For those who are already using their voice or words to communicate, music can support developing verbal skills by enhancing perception and encouraging vocal production. It can be especially potent if you have the support of a speech and language therapist (or are one).

Later chapters will discuss how we build skills that underpin and develop skills for speech, but before we consider why and how to use music to support verbal learning, we need to pause and imagine the musical world of learners like James. We begin our exploration with a big question: *how do people with learning differences perceive sound?* If we consider James, what was his sonic experience *like* as he played? How did his hearing loss affect what he heard; did his autism cause hypersensitivity to some sounds, or did it give him the ability to see, feel or taste the sounds he played? Did he attend to *all* sounds he heard at once or follow a single melody or timbre as it came and went? There is no ready answer to these questions. Unless we have a common language and the right words, we can only observe and infer what others hear, perceive or enjoy. However, we can gain some insight into the types of differences that James and others might experience by examining the nature of sound and why it affects us the way it does.

This chapter considers why sound and music have such an immediate and visceral impact on our bodies and emotions and explores how some learners might hear or perceive sound differently from you or me. In the first sections, I discuss the power of sound as music and therapy and introduce theories explaining why music can support language and speech. Next, I discuss the evidence that people with learning differences and developmental delays can develop musically. The chapter provides practical ideas that will help you think about how to begin working with sound and music with learners who cannot directly explain what they hear.

WHAT IS SOUND AND HOW DO WE SENSE IT?

In *physical terms*, sound is a vibration that travels through a medium. Vibration occurs when an object moves back and forth about a central point, displacing particles around it. These displaced particles bump into nearby particles, creating temporary dense clusters before moving back to their starting point, creating space (see Figure 1.1, and an example in Video 4 of the online resources). In this way, the vibrating object causes a pressure wave of high pressure (dense clusters of particles) and low pressure (low clusters of particles), which travels through the medium surrounding it (gas, liquid, solid). When the pressure wave hits a solid surface (such as the tympanic membrane, or eardrum), the surface begins to vibrate as the particles strike it. From the eardrum, the signal is passed via movement of the hammer (the 'stapes') to the fluid-filled cochlea; and from here, it passes as an electrical impulse to the brain (Figure 1.2).

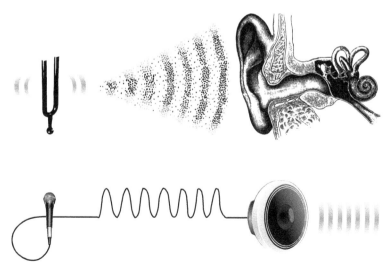

Figure 1.1: Sound is movement. The figure shows how the moving object (a tuning fork) causes air particles to move. These reach the ear where they strike the tympanic membrane, are converted to electrical impulses and sent to the auditory centre of the brain. If we hold a microphone to the tuning fork, the soundwave is transformed into an electrical signal and sent to a loudspeaker: the membrane of the speaker moves, setting in motion the air particles, which we hear in the same way as we hear the original sound.

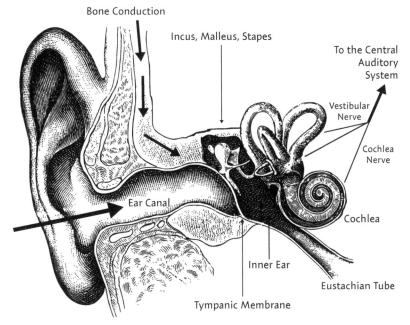

Figure 1.2: The anatomy of the ear, and the routes that sound takes towards the brain. Most people hear sound primarily via the ear canal, but some might receive a stronger signal via bone conduction. Note that there are two nerves marked: the cochlear nerve and the vestibular nerve. The vestibular nerve is associated with our sense of movement and balance.

When the electrical impulse reaches our brain, we perceive different qualities in the soundwave, such as volume and pitch. These qualities are physical in origin, but our understanding of them depends on our brain and body. The distance of movement of the object from its resting position is the *amplitude* – which we perceive as *loudness*. Our perception of *pitch* is related to how many times the object vibrates in a second (frequency, measured in Hertz). Although we measure frequency in seconds, the duration between each back-and-forth cycle could take nanoseconds or even years. As explained by Seth Horowitz (2012) in his book *The Universal Sense,* every vibration on Earth (and beyond) has the potential to be heard if we just had the right ears to hear. However, human ears can only detect a relatively limited range of frequency, and we each have our individual range within the possible spectrum of human hearing. Furthermore, our ears are optimized to hear vibrations in air, rather than – say – vibrations in liquids. However, we do also hear through solids: our own speech sounds, for example, are conducted to our auditory centre through bone, as well as through the airborne signal to our ear (see Figure 1.2). Our own physical properties lead to individual ways of hearing: each person we meet may have a different spectrum of hearing from us, may process more slowly or quickly than us, with greater or weaker definition, or may rely more on one form of sound conduction or medium than another.

Naturally, we emphasize the brain's ability to make sense of what we *hear*, but we should also consider the role of our *other senses*. The musicologist Nina Sun Eidsheim argues that the traditional description of sound as aural is limited. She believes that the vibrational properties lend themselves to more fully physical experiences and that we could explore sound transmission through alternative media, other than air. In her book *Sensing Sound,* Eidsheim (2015) discusses the experience of hearing opera through water, and of singing in water: the medium changes both what can be heard and the physical process of singing. When singing underwater with others, the feeling of the sound through body-to-body transmission became more important than hearing. I am not suggesting trying this: but almost every textbook on sound and hearing assumes that the *primary* medium of transmission is air. For some people, the auditory signal might be weak. For example, in people with hearing loss or with glue ear, the eustachian canal becomes blocked (see Figure 1.2) and can become inflamed; it is also common in people with Down syndrome or with cleft palate, for example. For these, the signal via bone conduction might be stronger and easier to perceive than the airborne signal.

Eidsheim also gives an example that makes us think about speech as *more than* sound. She gives an example of how we understand the speech sounds of /b/ (as in 'book') and /p/ (as in 'pick') as auditory events. In terms of physical properties, they each consist of the sudden release of air (movement) from closed, compressed lips; and, for /b/, we hear the soundwave that occurs when the vocal folds vibrate. However, Eidsheim argues that we can interpret these speech sounds as tactile sensations of air on skin. Taking her argument further, these speech sounds may be visual events, too, if we pay attention to how a speaker's lips move; or we might also feel the vibrations if we touch the larynx as we say the sounds. In other words, sound is multisensory.

In *psychological terms*, sounds – and music – can exist even in the absence of an external physical signal, or in an altered sensory form. The neuroscientist and author Oliver Sacks has reported on many people who hallucinate music (2007). In musical hallucinations, a person will hear music where none exists: as though it is playing in their room, or outside their window. This condition can prove more tenacious for some than the common *earworm*, persisting for months or years, even at volume. For some, these cases of musical hallucination resolve themselves spontaneously; or they reduce or fade with medication. For many, the causes of musical hallucinations remain mysterious, but some are linked to *hearing loss*: a case of the brain compensating for reduced stimulation. While musical hallucinations tend to persist, sound or music can be triggered temporarily by another sense, or sound might trigger another sense – a phenomenon termed synaesthesia. For example, the sight of a grapheme (letter or number) might trigger a tone or timbre, or sounds may trigger images, colours, scents or physical sensations. Scientists are not yet certain of the cause or causes of synaesthesia, but they believe it arises from a difference in brain architecture. It may be genetic, and is unusually common in people with autism (Baron-Cohen *et al.*, 2013).

The potential multisensory nature of sound is hugely important. It means we can draw on alternative ways of sensing sound to support children and young people in developing their music and early speech. For example, we might emphasize physical and visual properties of speech in teaching and therapy, by using techniques such as cued articulation, which captures the physical movements of speech sounds in visual form. Cued articulation can be especially powerful when coupled with short video clips that model articulatory movement of speech sounds (Lindley-Baker & Mills, 2022). We can remember, too, that some of these additional or alternative senses may be turned up or dialled down in some learners: they might not hear well through their ears, but they might be able to feel sound in their body, or on their skin. The entire argument of this book, and much of the science within it, rests on the fact that verbal communication and music are *auditory* events processed in the brain's auditory centres. This tenet is sound and practical, and the suggestions in the book are aimed at strengthening aural perception. Still, we must approach each child, young person and adult with openness to the fact that their experience may be individual and far removed from what we know or expect.

Sound and music are also closely related to our own physical *movement*. As infants, we instinctively move to music from birth, and our carers rock us and bounce us to songs and music. One of the social functions of music is that it lets us coordinate our movements with others to dance or work more efficiently. Music can also help people recover functional movements of limbs and speech after suffering brain damage. Music can help change the way we move, but the converse is also true: the way we move to music affects how we perceive the music. Just listening to music can prepare the brain for movement: for example, when pianists hear a piece they can play, or imagine the piece, their brains activate the motor systems in anticipation of making the physical movements (Taylor & Witt, 2015). This principle extends to speech movements, too: presenting the rhythms of words or phrases in a musical context primes the brain for the same rhythms in speech. Given that sound and music do not exist without movement, we must consider how and why some children move the way they do if we wish to support their ability to produce and control sound. This is a theme we will return to in each chapter.

SOUND, MIND AND BODY

Our perception of sound has an immediate and powerful effect on our *emotions*. The emotional power of sound can lie in the images and memories it provokes – for example, when the sound of the sea reminds us of a holiday, or a song triggers a memory of someone. But the auditory signal itself has a powerful effect below this cerebral level. The speed with which our brains process sound is so fast, and goes so quickly to the deepest centres of our brain, that sound can influence how we interpret what else we perceive (Horowitz, 2012). Film-makers and advertising companies exploit this emotional link: the internet is rife with examples of how the same scene can appear foreboding, thrilling, calm or comic, depending on its soundtrack. Most of all, the brain seeks pattern and rhythm in sound. Rhythm in nature keeps us in sync with our world: these natural rhythms may be simple, such as the burst-pause of noise and silence, or the loud-quiet swells that we hear in chorusing insects and the sounds of the sea. Tuning in to the rhythm in our environment keeps us safe: we are still primed to use our hearing to make sense of our environment and to monitor changes that may signal danger, even as we sleep. Rhythm is safe, reassuring: but sudden variation in our sonic environment can signal danger. When the singing of the birds stops, when alarm calls sound, our very physiology changes. We stop moving, we suspend our breath to focus, and our heart rate increases in preparation for fight or flight.

Music takes the power of sound and rhythm and adds punch. Music provides a reassuringly predictable structure that conveys a greater sense of safety than silence or ambient sound. As such, music can act as a screen or safety blanket against environmental stressors. Let us consider, for a moment, the number of children and young people who find their environment unpredictable and overwhelming, as James did. We can immediately see why allowing them to listen to their choice of music can reduce hypervigilance and anxious responses.

Music as therapy

The idea that music heals and transforms has a long pedigree. Historically, in early civilizations, music's power to heal has been associated with magic and ritual, often with the belief that 'disease' and 'disability' were rooted in emotional or spiritual causes. Evidence of music as therapy is found in documents from Ancient Egypt, China, Babylon and the Bible: skilled music healers could banish demons, appease the Gods, purge strong emotions, and aid physical and psychological healing: indeed, music was a power often ascribed to Gods and gifted mortals, such as Orpheus, who could use music to move the Earth itself. In Ancient Greece, for example, the teachings of Pythagoras and Damon inspired musical prescriptions and educational programmes to keep the body and mind healthy. Certain modes or musical scales, akin to the major and minor scales still used in Western music, were recommended for different activities. Pythagoreans recommended one mode at the start of the day, to energize; one to foster feelings of strength and courage; and another mode to unwind at the day's end (West, 1992). Neuroscientists have since confirmed how powerful music can be, and why. Our preferred music taps into our emotions and our bodies; when we listen to music we like, our brains are flooded with chemicals that make us feel good. Our heart rate and our blood pressure change, depending on the type and tempo of the music (Levitin, 2006). These physiological effects energize and calm us, just as our ancestors believed.

Exciting developments in technology show how the body-music link may offer insights into our emotional states: measurements of the body's electrophysiological signals – heart rate, skin conductance, respiration rate – can be converted into sound. These sounds – referred to as *biomusic* – can be used to alter the physiological state, and offer an alternative way to communicate and build connections. Such technology can open up new channels for people who do not or cannot directly identify what they feel or express their feelings in sound (Blain-Moraes *et al.*, 2013).

However, no special equipment is needed to use music as a tool that supports emotional connection and communication. Craig and Lisa, who both work as psychologists, explain how they and their daughter, Annie, benefit from making music:

Our daughter was born with multiple needs, including epilepsy, communication needs, spastic quadriplegia, visual issues and learning needs. My wife and I have applied ideas that we are familiar with associated with psychology, special needs and developmental neurology to help support all three of us over the years. Our daughter is now 16 years old.

Professionally, we know how important early development is for all children. For our daughter, we saw music, rhyme, rhythm, songs and instruments as a way to supplement her life. We would use songs to create routine at the start and end of activities. We saw singing as a method to make dialogue predictable and familiar. When considering mood, we used songs and recordings to create times for calm and for excitement.

A key element of our journey together has been the application and use of sound and music. From before birth, and from a very young age, we used rhyme, music and sound to help build some predictability and focus for our daughter. We found that songs helped in managing her high levels of emotional arousal and helped her regulate her sensory needs. Music enabled us to play listening games, signal times of the day, better manage transitions and create positive interactions.

Creating interaction and turn-taking with a young person who finds movement, focus and speech very, very difficult may be a challenge. We looked towards music and sound as a way to develop those experiences and skills; we would use volume, style, rhythm and tone to help our daughter feel she could contribute and engage in social exchange.

Now our daughter is much older we continue to use music to support her. Our home has become a place of music. When we have visitors, we have percussion instruments and encourage everyone to join in with singing, listening and playing along together. On our calendar, we have live music activities that we attend and these are some of the most eagerly anticipated events in our daughter's life. Music and sound have become positive and fun tools to help us come together and create a common framework for interaction with family and friends.

As we have grown together, we have found that music has helped to share activities with a range of people and we have made new friends and connections. Our daughter's love of music has widened the range of music that we, as her parents, listen to and enjoy. What we have seen is that sound activities and music enable all to participate; they create inclusion, emotions and positive memories.

Craig, Lisa and Annie

MUSIC, LANGUAGE AND SPEECH

Language remains a key area of difficulty throughout the lives of many children, especially if they have quite complex or overlapping needs. Language is a complex symbolic system. If spoken or written, it includes words and the rules that govern their use (syntax), register and semantics (meaning). Speech is concerned with the physical production of sounds, words and phrases; and the communication of meaning via word choice and paraverbal signals, such as tone of voice, pitch and rhythm. It can take any child years to master these complexities, sometimes decades; but we can begin to strengthen the skills that support music and verbal learning from the moment they are born.

MUSICAL BEGINNINGS

Imagine a typically developing baby in its mother's womb, at about 20 weeks of gestation. Its environment is quiet and muted but rich in sensory information, and the baby can feel something of the world it will be born into. Secure in its dark, watery world, the baby is rocked by its mother's footsteps and feels the rhythmic pulse of her heart beating a steady pulse of life through both their bodies. The soundscape of the womb is diverse: a diffuse background noise of blood flow, breathing and movements is punctuated by the noise of people, televisions, traffic. These soundwaves travel through the amniotic fluid and push against the membrane of the baby's developing ear drum. The moving membrane sets in motion the tiny bones of the middle ear, which tap on the cochlea, amplify the sound and ripple the fluid of the inner ear. These ripples disperse like waves on a reed-filled pond: the passing of each wave bends bundled hairs that sit atop the tens of thousands of nerves, triggering electrical waveforms that reach the area of the brain that will specialize in processing sound. About this time, four months before the baby is born, these hearing systems mature just enough for the developing baby to hear as well as feel its mother's heart and her voice. The baby feels the motion of an in-breath pull upwards on its mother's diaphragm; it feels her voice as it resonates in her upper body and conducts the vibrations, via tissue and bone, to its own body; almost simultaneously, it hears parts of the airborne vocal signal as it moves through the walls of her belly and through the amniotic fluid. This voice carries sounds that cut through the background noise and add to the tangible, bone-conducted buzz: soft muted vowels, the stop-start of syllables, rising and falling melodies; new sounds mixing with old familiar sounds.

The filtered sounds of the womb prime us for language learning and give the newborn something familiar and reassuring to connect with when they emerge into the unfamiliar, bright new world. Newly born, we use our in-utero learning to tune in to our immediate environment, and to be tuned by it. We use the rhythms of our mother's speech, familiar from our final four months in the womb, to pick out our mother-tongue from the richer sonic world and to latch on to its rhythmic patterns and contrasting timbres.

The newborn uses the musical elements of language to make sense of their auditory world and seek comfort and connection with others. Colwyn Trevarthen, a renowned child development and psychology expert, cites an astonishing example of a five-month old baby, born blind, who conducted her mother as she sang a song. The infant's gestures expressed the melodic and rhythmic phrases of the song, and were timed *just ahead* of her mother's voice. Trevarthen argues that the child's response derives from an 'intrinsic motive pulse', an innate ability to produce sensorimotor movement to an internal clock:

This is an extraordinarily important case for the science of psychology, because it shows how the motive pulse, the IMP, in the baby, directing activity in muscles of her arm and hand, 'hears' the mother. It assimilates the message heard in the movements of the mother's musical vocal system and feeds them to the rhythms of the baby's hand waiving [sic] in a space of melody imagined around her body. Her hand points up to her head as her mother's voice rises in pitch, and drops at the wrist at the close of a stanza, just like the gestures that would be made by a trained conductor who is leading an orchestra. We have to accept that this is a pure innate intuition for the impulse of music, because the baby has never seen her own hands move, nor anyone else's. She feels the music in her being and moves to let it out. (Trevarthen, 2008, p.27)

This example illustrates how sound and movement are connected, instinctively, and how we use musical-movement gestures to interact. Trevarthen stresses that most babies and carers engage in a similarly subconscious dance, in which the baby's gestures match the syllable patterns of their carer (2008). He also points out that these movements are very early language: they are a narrative form and syntax. From birth, we learn to share experiences using short 'phrases' of movement, sound and emotional expression long before we form the sounds that become words. For all of us, music is our first language.

MUSIC, LANGUAGE AND THE BRAIN

Our 'first' language of music can be more easily perceived, processed and learned than verbal language. Furthermore, as a growing body of scientific evidence shows, music can be used to support and develop the skills we need for spoken language. Studies of musicians' brains confirm that their brains are much better at processing sound, in general, than non-musicians, and that some of these skills can benefit language (for reviews, see Besson, Chobert & Marie, 2011; Kraus & Chandrasekaran, 2010). Music and language share similar properties, such as phrasing, pitch, rhythm and timbre; and they also share cognitive processes, such as attention to sound, memory for sound, and pattern recognition. Music training can improve some of these skills, leading to better musicianship and better language abilities. Children who have undertaken musical training outperform their non-musician peers in cognitive skills that underpin language learning, such as auditory memory and executive function (Zuk, *et al.,* 2014). They also have superior auditory abilities, including: enhanced processing of pitch patterns, lexical stress, metrical structure of words, and speech in noise; faster processing of variation in rhythm pitch and harmony; and more accurate reading skills. Recently, some studies confirm that music training can cause these changes (e.g. Habibi *et al.*, 2018; Frischen, Schwarzer & Degé, 2021). In such studies, the children did not take up music because they were *already* good with sound.

Some theorists agree that learning to play an instrument can support verbal language when specific conditions are met during musical practice. The OPERA hypothesis (Patel, 2011, 2014) was proposed to explain how skills in music learning can transfer to the language domain when certain conditions are met. The hypothesis outlines five main conditions: overlap (O) in the neural resources used for music and for language (i.e. the music-making must use some of the same areas of the brain and its neurological networks as language); for skills to transfer, the player must perform with greater precision (P) in music than is needed for language; they must gain emotional reward (E); repeat (R) the activity; and play with sustained attention (A).

After further research by scientists studying music, language and cognition, Patel revised the hypothesis to the 'expanded' version (2014). The later version added that music could drive change in language if a sensory process (e.g. encoding frequency or rhythm) or a cognitive process (such as memory) shared brain networks when being used for music and language. The expanded hypothesis argues that transfer to language takes place if music training places greater demands on these brain networks and processes than are needed for language – that is, music training will require greater awareness and precision of timing and pitch, and will place greater demands on memory for sound; and at the same time, the learner must be engaged, attentive and must find enjoyment in it. As we will see in later chapters, we can adapt musical activities to keep the learner engaged and challenged, while also encouraging precision, practice and learning. We will revisit the extended theory in Chapter 10. But now, let us consider how far music might transfer in learners with additional or complex needs, and what other factors we might consider to support this process.

HOW CAN MUSIC BENEFIT PEOPLE WITH ADDITIONAL OR COMPLEX LEARNING NEEDS?

There is no reason to think that children, young people or adults with complex learning needs cannot benefit from music in the same ways we all can. Like James or Annie, the majority will benefit from making music simply because it gives them pleasure. Add to this the evidence that music can support wellbeing and aid communication and social bonding, and the real argument becomes: why would you NOT do music? However, if we ask *to what extent will music benefit their verbal skills* or *will making music help my child to speak*, the answer is more complex. The similarities between music and speech are much closer than between music and language, and the 'transfer' distance is shorter: indeed, if we use songs and singing as a teaching tool, the transfer of skills is 'within-domain', rather than 'cross-domain' (Patel, 2014).

Studies show that music-making can support language development in some children and adults with communication differences (e.g. Vaiouli & Andreou, 2018; Torppa & Huotilainen, 2019), but many children and young people are not yet at the stage of developing language, for multiple reasons. There is a lack of rigorous experiment-based research evidence regarding the possible transfer of skills from music to speech in people with learning differences or complex learning needs. However, the types of people we are thinking about in this book might benefit more from music than children with better language skills. They are still learning some of the foundational skills that are common to music and speech. Indeed, a recent systematic review by Swaminathan and Schellenberg (2020) examined the claims that rhythm training could lead to language improvements; although they found flaws with many claims, they agreed that studies involving children who have dyslexia (Flaugnacco *et al.*, 2015) and hearing loss (Hidalgo, Falk & Schön, 2017) were robust. They proposed that those with delays and differences in language might benefit from music-making more than children with milder language impairments. However, they stressed that training may need to be more intensive to be effective.

Before any skill transfers from music to the language domain, there needs to be progress in musical ability. This leads us to our final question: *what progress can people make in music if they have atypical learning needs and developmental pathways?*

Musicality in people with learning differences and disabilities

So far, we have explored the possibility that some of the learners you will work with may have different sound experiences than you expect. For some, these differences may have begun in the womb, for example from minor changes in the ear, auditory pathways and networks, or the central nervous system. From birth, any small differences will be magnified: consequently, their journey towards both music and speech will have been different from our own from before the moment they were born. Therefore, we must expect that some of the young people we work with will process information differently from the way we expect; they may have altered brain functioning and processing speeds and different rates of learning. Currently, there is no research to help us understand how the earliest musical experiences of children with additional needs compare to those of a typically developing child. However, there is evidence that most learners with developmental, learning and sensory differences do learn to enjoy and make music, and can develop their skills. For many, music is something they can excel at, especially as it does not require language. Some learners, like James, have heightened *musicality* – a term that signifies sensitivity to music as well as musical ability and musical learning (Houlahan & Tacka, 2015). Some go on to perform at professional levels, like the pianist Derek Paravicini, who was born blind, with autism and learning difficulties (Ockelford, 2013).

A few key studies have examined musical ability or development in people with different levels of cognitive ability. Research by Ockelford *et al.* (2011) and the Sounds of Intent project (http://soundsofintent.org) confirms that children with complex and profound learning disabilities can develop musically. Over six months, teachers and researchers charted the development of 20 adolescents (aged 11–17 years) who took part in weekly 45-minute sessions of song-based musical activity. The pupils made progress in listening and responding, causing, creating and controlling sound, and interaction. Although the authors attributed much of the group's rapid development to increased confidence and familiarity for the staff and pupils alike, the data showed an ability for learners to develop. This adds to earlier evidence from MacDonald, O'Donnell and Davies (1999), who considered the educational and therapeutic value of musical activities for 20 people with mild to moderate learning disabilities, aged 17–58 years. The intervention group received training in playing the gamelan; one control group received training in cooking and art; and a second control group did not receive additional training. Each group was tested before and after the intervention periods on rhythm production and pitch perception, and on the Communication Assessment Profile for Adults with Mental Handicap (CASP). All programmes ran once a week for ten weeks. The music group made statistically significant improvements in measures of imitating simple rhythms (clapping), instrumental rhythms, and in section 3 of CASP, which measures pragmatic communication, and involved picture identification and picture-naming tasks.

Although scientific studies are rare, learners with complex and varied needs can progress in their musical skills. However, we must understand the challenges and barriers that some young people face in different areas of music learning. The remaining chapters in this book will help you understand some of these differences. They offer practical guidance for adapting musical activities so you can support learners and enhance the likelihood of transfer of learning from music to speech.

CONCLUSIONS

Let us return to the beginning and reconsider how people with learning differences perceive sound. We may never know what the sonic world of another is like, but we can be open to the idea that it is different from our own. This gives us some ideas to consider when doing musical activities with them. For example:

- What sounds do they like, and which do they avoid? Consider sounds in the environment, not just musical sounds: water dripping, phones chiming, paper rustling, wind...
- How do they respond to simple sounds (tones) and complex tones (chords); to harmony or discord?
- Do they favour one ear over another? Does their hearing (or listening ability) seem to fluctuate?
- What sounds do they make?
- What volume do they respond to best?
- Do they seem to need to limit their auditory input?
- How do they respond to feeling or seeing sound instead of hearing it?

The activities in the following chapters focus on supporting movement to sound and awareness of sound, using music-making activities. If we can help learners become more aware and precise as they move, sing and listen, these skills may extend to verbal learning. But for some children, the first step may be to explore sound itself. The starting place may even be with exploring silence: one of my young students played an empty egg shaker for months; he then progressed to a beanbag that rustled when he played it, and later to a cabasa. Although our focus is on sound, the appeal of other senses and textures can be just as helpful in learning to make musical movements.

Finding out about your young person's hearing abilities will help you identify which sounds are more accessible to them, both in terms of musical sounds and speech sounds. Where possible, seek advice from audiologists, speech and language therapists or other specialist providers who can support you in understanding the sonic world the child inhabits.

CHAPTER SUMMARY

For all of us, sound can be a powerful means of connecting with others, with or without language. In musical forms, especially, sound can have powerful physiological and emotional effects: it can change how we feel in our bodies, and how safe we feel in our environment. However, sound – and therefore music – has psychological properties as well as physical properties; our own bodies and brains determine how each of us hears, processes and responds to the same sound. Each of us will have a different response to the 'same' sound; for learners whose brains and bodies are not like our own, we may need to explore sound and music carefully, and be alert to our differences. It is important to be cautious in monitoring responses, especially in people who have limited means of self-expression, or whose physical and sensory needs are different from our own. For those who enjoy the sounds and music we can offer them, we can begin to explore how to use music to cause changes – if we begin to develop skills in listening, in musical motor-timing and singing, we will be encouraging the related areas of the brain to 'grow' and connect and get better at working with sound and movement. Although we cannot predict how far the ripples will spread, we can be confident we are strengthening the skills that underpin verbal learning by supporting the learner's musicality.

RECOMMENDED READING

Horowitz, S.S. (2012). *The Universal Sense: How Hearing Shapes the Mind*. New York, NY: Bloomsbury Publishing.

Levitin, D.J. (2006). *This is Your Brain on Music: The Science of a Human Obsession*. New York, NY: Penguin.

Ockelford, A. (2013). *Music, Language and Autism: Exceptional Strategies for Exceptional Minds*. London: Jessica Kingsley Publishers.

Sacks, O. (2010). *Musicophilia: Tales of Music and the Brain*. Toronto: Vintage Canada.

PART 1

Rhythm Skills

CHAPTER 2

Finding the Heartbeat of Music and Speech

THE BIG QUESTIONS

Why is the beat important for verbal learning? How can I help young people become better at moving in time to the beat?

By the end of this chapter, you will know:

- what skills are involved in being able to detect and synchronize (entrain) to a beat
- how skills in entrainment relate to verbal learning
- how and why some people have difficulties in matching movements to a beat
- how to support beat perception and production in learners who are at different developmental stages.

WHO IS THIS FOR?

This chapter is of interest to anyone wishing to use music to support developing speech perception.

It is of relevance to people who work with individuals with *Down syndrome* and *sensory processing disorders*, including some *auditory processing disorders (APD)*, *autism*, *ADHD*, *cerebral palsy*, *dyslexia*, *dyspraxia* and *hearing impairments*.

We find rhythm in the macro and micro levels of life. We see it in the ebb and flow of seas; the cycle of day and night; or feel it in the beating of our hearts and the rise and fall of our breath. Such rhythms are formed of patterns that repeat over time – dark versus light, noise versus silence. There is a predictability to rhythmic cycles in nature, but the patterns do not need to repeat exactly. In music, though, we require a level of rhythm that is as close to periodical as possible. This is often called an *isochronous* rhythm – that is, the duration between sounds is equal. In less formal literature, isochrony is called the *pulse* or the *beat*.

The ability to perceive and play a steady beat or pulse is the foundation of rhythm in music; its predictable cycle enables us to move, sing and play in time with each other. As we will explore, the ability to perceive a steady beat connects closely with language perception and literacy and with a broader range of communicative skills that underpin verbal communication. This chapter will explain the links between rhythmic pulse, movement and verbal learning. It will explain why the perception of the pulse is valuable for verbal learning. It will discuss why some people may have difficulty perceiving and synchronizing to a beat in music and suggest how you might strengthen and develop beat awareness and precision in young people. This chapter also sets the foundation for Chapter 3, which explores the links between rhythm (non-isochronous) in music and rhythm in communication and speech; and Chapter 4, which explores the nature of spoken and musical rhythm difficulties in people with speech difficulties.

MOVEMENT, ENTRAINMENT AND VOCAL LEARNING

Our brains are wired for rhythmic movement. This brain function enables even 'simple' animals, such as worms, to move within their environment and breathe. Some animals can synchronize their movements to an external source. This allows them to act together to create rhythms in movement, sound or vision. Hence, a lizard or bird might bob its head in synchrony with another, and the calls of insects and frogs may coincide. This ability to synchronize requires certain conditions to be met. Before an animal can synchronize to an externally produced signal, the signal itself needs to be *isochronous* – that is, there will be an equal duration between each sound, motion or flash. The animal needs a brain that can perceive the incoming signal, predict the next signal, align its movements precisely to the signal, and monitor and adjust the timing of its actions.

This ability to synchronize is found across the animal kingdom and serves various social and communicative purposes. For example, when frogs and insects closely synchronize their calls, and male fireflies flash in perfect time, they amplify the signal to attract mates or deter predators. However, entrainment to an *auditory* signal, such as music, is rare in animals; among primates, it is unique to humans (Merchant & Honing, 2014). While some primates, such as macaques, can be trained to produce a regular beat, they move in response to the beat that has *just gone*, rather than predicting when the next beat will fall. As a result, they cannot entrain to music: entrainment requires us to predict the next beat so that we raise our hand or foot far enough in advance that it *falls* on the next beat. Only a handful of non-human animals spontaneously move or dance to music – to date, these include zebra finches; parrots, which can synchronize and adapt to a range of tempi; some elephants and a sea lion (see Honing, 2019). Entrainment occurs primarily in vocal animals. This observation has prompted suggestions that musical synchrony has a close relationship with vocal learning (e.g. Patel, 2021), but this theory is not yet proven.

In contrast to most animals, humans respond instinctively to music through movement. When young babies hear music, they kick their legs or beat their arms. As children and adults, we might tap our feet or nod our heads without even being conscious that we are doing so. Keeping to the beat is essential in most cultural forms of music – a steady, predictable pulse helps musicians play in time with each other, and enables musical notes to coincide perfectly with one another, thereby creating melodies, harmonies or discord. While hearing and moving to a beat is essential for musicians, it is also important to us as social animals. A tangible beat helps us coordinate our movements with other people when dancing or working. Doing so strengthens social bonds, making us feel more 'at one' with each other.

HOW DOES BEAT ENTRAINMENT RELATE TO VERBAL DEVELOPMENT AND LANGUAGE?
Rhythm and rise time

Accuracy in moving to the beat is linked to phonological skills – detecting syllables, sounds and rhyme in verbal language. We know this because many people with speech or language difficulties, such as *developmental language disorder* (DLD) or *dyslexia*, have trouble matching movements to a beat (see Leong & Goswami, 2014; Roche *et al.*, 2016). Their difficulties in beat entrainment and language are believed to stem from a difference in the part of their brains that detects or integrates changes in how a sound's energy changes over time (Goswami, 2019a). In music, for example, the spectral envelope is the change in energy and timbre that helps us distinguish a violin from a drum. In speech, these types of changes help us differentiate phonemes and syllables: when we speak the sound

/b/ (as in 'book'), it produces a different sound spectrum than a /p/ (as in 'paper'), for example. Specifically, some groups of people seem to have problems perceiving *'rise time'*, which is the *rate* at which the sound energy changes. In speech, the rise-time is the duration between the onset of the first speech sound in a syllable to the peak amplitude of the vowel. The rise time depends on linguistic characteristics, such as how we emphasize some words or sounds, and on articulatory factors, such as consonant and vowel combinations. For example, as Figure 2.1 shows, the rise time is different between onset and vowel in the words sit, spit and split. The images show how the change from onset to mid-vowel is much faster (a steeper rise) in 'sit', and lengthens as more sounds are introduced.

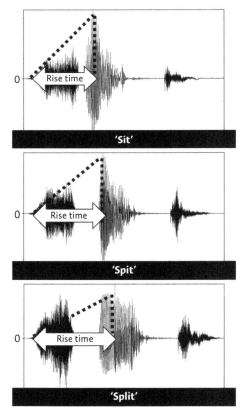

Figure 2.1: Rise time in single-syllable words. The rise time is defined as the rate at which the spoken sound reaches peak amplitude between the onset of the word and the first vowel. In the figures above, the sound envelope is represented by the slope of the triangle; the bottom line of the triangle represents the rise time. The base line is shortest in 'sit', representing faster changes in sound energy. The more complex sounds in 'spit' and 'split' take longer to articulate, affecting the rise time.

Rhythm in speech and music

The ability to perceive peaks in sound energy is common to music and speech, and it is essential in helping us keep track of time. When playing an instrument or singing, our ability to synchronize depends on us matching the peak energy of our sound (a note or a syllable) to the peak energy of another sound (e.g. the beat). In music, the stronger beats help us perceive 'hierarchies' of beat and meter (see Figure 2.2). Try tapping along to a piece of music you know well: notice your own preferred tapping rate – but you can also tap at twice the rate, or half the rate.

Conversational speech has no pulse, but some forms of speech are strongly rhythmic, such as poetry and rhyme. Say the rhyme 'Humpty Dumpty' and feel its rhythm; notice what you do to emphasize the stronger sounds. Below, you can see how the rhythm changed when I said 'Humpty Dumpty sat on a wall' (Figure 2.3a), and when I spoke about it (Figure 2.3b). In the rhyme, there is a sense of a 3/4 meter (waltz time); whereas there is no meter when I talk, and the duration between syllables is more variable. Notice, too, how the pitch is higher and the intensity is greater (louder) on the stressed syllables. To learn more, see Video 1 in the online resources.

We will revisit accent and stress in sound in Chapter 3, when we discuss rhythm and the role of the syllable, in particular. For now, it is enough to understand that both beat entrainment and verbal language learning depend on our ability to hear and track energy changes in sound. Without this ability, we might not perceive the pulse of music, rhythm in speech or the subtle changes that help us tell apart similar sounds or syllables. In verbal learning, this difficulty has consequences for linking sounds to symbols: if someone cannot track the changes in sound well enough to perceive the phoneme or syllable or word, they cannot link that sound to its written form. The connection between verbal development and beat entrainment is so strong that tapping ability can predict skills in reading, speech and language across many languages and writing systems. It is also strong enough that learning to tap or play in time to music changes how the brain perceives speech sounds, and can improve phonological skills.

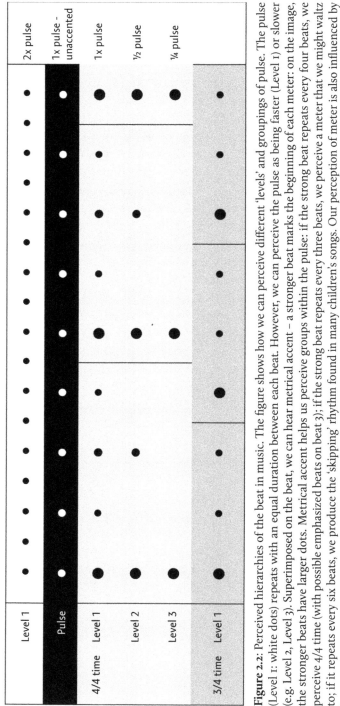

Figure 2.2: Perceived hierarchies of the beat in music. The figure shows how we can perceive different 'levels' and groupings of pulse. The pulse (Level 1: white dots) repeats with an equal duration between each beat. However, we can perceive the pulse as being faster (Level 1) or slower (e.g. Level 2, Level 3). Superimposed on the beat, we can hear metrical accent – a stronger beat marks the beginning of each meter: on the image, the stronger beats have larger dots. Metrical accent helps us perceive groups within the pulse: if the strong beat repeats every four beats, we perceive 4/4 time (with possible emphasized beats on beat 3); if the strong beat repeats every three beats, we perceive a meter that we might waltz to; if it repeats every six beats, we produce the 'skipping' rhythm found in many children's songs. Our perception of meter is also influenced by how we dance or move to a beat.

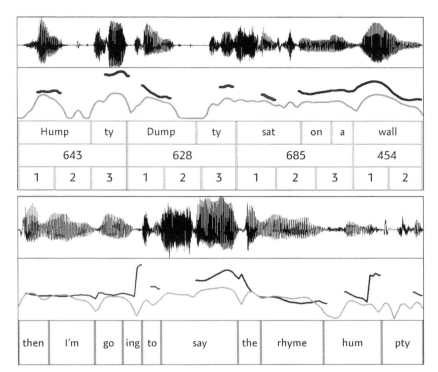

Figure 2.3: Rhythm of speech and rhyme. The figure shows an extract of the rhyme, 'Humpty Dumpty' (Figure 2.3a, top image), and conversational speech (Figure 2.3b, lower image). The rhyme has a strong rhythmic feel (in waltz time), created in part by changes in pitch and amplitude, and by the consistency in duration between accented syllables. In contrast, the duration varies between successive syllables when I talk about the rhyme: the emphasized word 'say' has longer duration, higher pitch and higher intensity than unaccented syllables. Note: there are complex interactions between pitch, intensity, duration and articulation that influence our perception of syllable boundaries. You can learn more about this in Video 1 in the online resources.

WHY DO SOME PEOPLE HAVE DIFFICULTIES PERCEIVING THE BEAT?

In practice, some people face multiple challenges in perceiving the subtle temporal cues that underpin both beat entrainment and speech. Many children and young adults, especially those with developmental delays, have comorbid conditions that can interact with each other, exacerbating any difficulties in perception, cognition or movement. For example, a child may have *hearing loss* and *auditory processing difficulties*, which will both affect perception; they may also have differences in how their *memory* retains, processes, retrieves and stores information;

they may have problems in sustaining or switching *attention* to different sensory stimuli, especially in noisy environments such as the classroom; and they may have *motor* or *cognitive differences* that affect the range, speed and accuracy of motor movements. The case studies of Chloe and Georgina, below, will help explain and contextualize these differences. The case studies help us understand what challenges are faced by someone with comorbid difficulties and help us consider how to reduce barriers to learning. If we can address challenges and reduce barriers to learning, we can help learners develop more accurate beat timing. Given the close connection between beat timing and perception of speech sounds (and possibly language and reading), it is essential to develop these foundational skills in music and motor-timing if music is to have a more comprehensive benefit for speech.

COMPLEX CASES

Case study: Chloe

Chloe is a cheerful, small, blond-haired young adult of 18 years. She has a big smile and loves to dance, sing and spend time with her friends. Like many people with Down syndrome, she has hearing loss in both ears. And like many young adults, she won't wear hearing aids and never has. Hearing loss can make it difficult for people like Chloe to hear some speech sounds, especially the quick, high-frequency sounds like 's', 'sh' and 'f'. Hearing loss also makes it hard for her to hear her voice, which is relatively high in pitch and quite 'whispery' for her age. It can be tough to understand Chloe when she is speaking and singing because she has not learned some speech sounds and has difficulty forming the sounds she uses.

Although Chloe likes music and dancing, she needs help to match her movements to the beat of the music. If she uses only her ears to guide her, her movements seem slow and delayed. If asked to copy actions, she can also be slow to respond and appear uncoordinated. She seems unsure of her balance and can become unsteady unless she can see her feet. Chloe's difficulties in moving in time to music are unsurprising for many reasons, including differences in how her muscles work and how well she perceives sound and movement. Like other people with Down syndrome, Chloe has some underdeveloped or weak muscles. Her hypermobility, ligamentous laxity and low muscle tone make controlled movement more difficult. While having lax ligaments gives her a good range of motion, her movements can be unstable and imprecise. In addition, her hypermobility can make it more difficult for her to know where her limbs are when she cannot see them – such as her feet.

Chloe's hearing impairment further complicates things. Hearing is linked to our ability to balance – as you will know if you have had a head cold or similar that has affected your balance. Hearing loss means that the signal reaching Chloe's brain is missing information. It can also mean that the signal reaches her brain more slowly or that the signal is reduced in quality. This combination of physical factors makes it very hard for Chloe to respond quickly and accurately to sounds – she must pay close attention to too many things at once that most of us take for granted.

To perceive a beat, we rely on an ability to process changes in sound energy. However, we need to use physiological and cognitive processes to move in time to that beat when tapping a foot, banging a drum or singing a song. To synchronize with accuracy, we need the auditory motor and auditory feedback systems to work closely together, and we require precise motor timing. Let us use Chloe as an example of these processes in action. The process below is illustrated in Figure 2.4. Assuming that she hears the beat, if Chloe wants to move in time to the beat, the following chain of events must happen:

1. Her brain needs to register the time difference between beats – for example, in a beat of 120 bpm (beats per minute), the time interval between beats is 500 ms, or half a second.
2. After hearing a few beats, Chloe unconsciously creates a 'template' of the pattern and holds it in auditory memory (Figure 2.4). This allows her to anticipate when the next beat will happen and plan her movement. As adults, we can usually do this by hearing just two beats, but Chloe's hearing loss means that she might need to hear more repetitions before forming the template.
3. To synchronize her movements to the beat, the auditory motor system of Chloe's brain needs to instruct the relevant muscles to move *before* the next beat so that this movement – be it a tap, clap, stamp or step – coincides with the beat.
4. She will need to receive feedback to check if the duration between

her movements was equal to the duration of the signal and if the sound she produced was in time with the input – to do this, she needs to notice whether the sound she made or the movement that she felt occurred before, after or on time with the beat.

5. Using the auditory feedback from her ears and tactile and motor feedback from her body, she will be able to adjust her limb movements. She will initiate her action sooner if she notices her tapping lagged behind the beat; or add more time if her previous movement preceded the beat. The sequence then repeats from point 3. These processes happen quickly and at a subconscious level. They can be harder for people like Chloe, who has hearing loss, frequent glue ear, a weak auditory memory, and difficulties in motor planning or motor coordination.

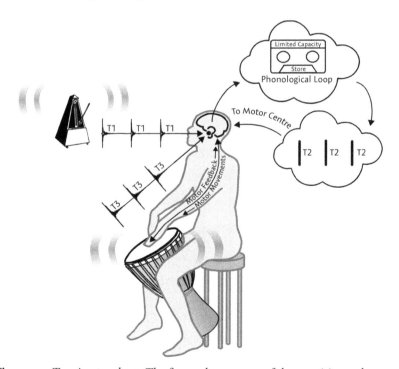

Figure 2.4: Tapping to a beat. The figure shows some of the cognitive and sensory processes that we use when we tap to an audible beat. The metronome is heard and temporarily stored in the phonological loop – a notional part of working memory that has a limited capacity for sound. It temporarily holds the pattern and the brain calculates the duration between successive taps, enabling us to form a 'template'. This template is used to plan our motor movements so that we tap the drum with the correct duration (T) between successive taps. The diagram shows how we use sensory feedback from our ears and body to monitor our tapping.

These types of difficulties are common in children and adults with many types of need, as well as Down syndrome. They each will need a little extra help to perceive the move in time to a beat.

I will now introduce another young adult and compare her skills in beat timing with Chloe's. Georgina and Chloe are similar in many ways: they are the same age, had similar experiences in school and college, have Down syndrome, and are both described as having 'severe' learning disabilities. However, they have contrasting music skills that arise from physical, cognitive and experiential differences. This comparison helped me understand some of the difficulties that individuals with complex learning needs, such as Down syndrome, might have in making music, and some of the factors and approaches that can help, which I will explain later in the chapter.

Case study: Chloe and Georgina

Chloe chooses a hand-held drum, about 10 inches in diameter, and a beater with a foam grip on one end, to make it easier to use. She chooses a song to play from her CD collection and drums along, singing simultaneously. Her movements are imprecise – some fall in the middle of the drum, some hit the frame. Her timing is erratic, especially when she sings, with her drumbeats falling behind those on the CD. I want to learn more about her ability to synchronize – or entrain – to a beat, so I make things a little easier for her. I play her a sequence of drumbeats, evenly spaced at 120 bpm, and ask her to tap along on the drum using her hand. The drum pattern is programmed at a medium tempo to start with; then it gets faster; then it gets slower. A few things are clear to me: despite Chloe's moderate hearing loss and refusal to wear a hearing aid, I know she can hear the beat because she changes her tempo when the drum pattern changes, without me telling her to. However, she cannot make her movements match the beat independently. When I give her a visual cue, by tapping with her and telling her to watch, she does much better. When I look at the recordings later, I also learn that she is more accurate when the tempo is fast than when it is slow.

Let's now turn to Georgina. Georgina has a small degree of hearing loss, but she has not been tested for years. No one seems to know how much it affects her. She seems to hear speech when it is directed at her, with no need to raise the volume. Georgina loves music, especially rock music. She has had drumming lessons once a week on a complete drum kit, where she plays Queen and ABBA and other pieces of music she takes along. When I give her the frame drum and beater and ask her to play along to music, she finds the beat immediately. When I ask her to tap to the simple beat, I do not tell her that the tempo will change suddenly, and she notices immediately and adjusts her tapping. When I look at the recording, I can see that her drumming is very close to the recorded pattern at fast, medium and slow tempi. In fact, sometimes, it is perfectly aligned.

As Georgina's ability to synchronize to a beat is so good, I give her an extra challenge: can she sing a song that she has just learned and show me the beat on a drum by tapping it as she sings? This is an advanced musical skill – it requires the brain to divide attention between different activities. For example, Georgina must plan ahead how fast she will sing and play; she must time her taps to match the first beat of each phrase she sings; she must simultaneously recall the words, the rhythm of the words, and the melody; she must simultaneously coordinate her voice and oro-motor movements with her breath, and coordinate her arm movements for tapping; and she must receive and monitor feedback from her ears and her hand movements to keep everything in sync. This places significant demands on her memory and on the parts of her brain that manage motor movements and self-awareness. For short bursts, she can do it all.

Georgina and Chloe have much in common but are at different levels regarding their ability to move to the beat. The following section explores some reasons for this difference. It will consider how we can use the information to support the ability to match movements to a beat and why this matters for speech.

What can we learn from Chloe and Georgina?
Georgina and Chloe differ in their drumming experience and their hearing abilities. We all need experience in the form of practice if we wish to develop a skill. However, several unusual features of Chloe's playing tell me that her hearing loss is the most significant factor: more so than her poor motor coordination.

First, Chloe's movements when tapping to a beat at any tempo were *irregular*. When I gave her a visual demonstration to focus on, she was able to make more regular movements – this clarifies that she does not have difficulty making rhythmic *movements*, so there must be a differ-ent explanation. Chloe's beats also typically came *after the beat*. This is unusual: most people can form a mental template that helps them to make their move micro-seconds ahead of the target beat. Georgina was very good at this. Playing after the beat suggests that Chloe reacts to the beat rather than predicts it. Possibly, this is caused by *poor coupling between auditory information and motor response* (Thaut, 2005). That is, the sensory signals from her ears and body do not arrive in Chloe's brain simultaneously, preventing smooth integration. Suppose we imagine that the sound from Chloe's drum as it reaches her auditory cortex arrives at a different time from the physical and visual sense of hitting the drum and from the sound of the beat on the recording. In that case, we can see that it is difficult for her to work out when to hit the drum. The 'pattern' that she plays is distorted and unclear because she has no clear mental representation of the pattern itself. For us, this distortion may be likened to how we perceive thunder and lightning as separate effects: in reality, they co-occur, but the sound of thunder can take much longer to reach us. Like thunder and lightning, Chloe's brain might receive signals at different points in time: consequently, entrainment is a significant challenge for Chloe, if not impossible.

Another difference between Georgina and Chloe is that Chloe's per-formance improved when she played fast. Chloe's ability to play more accurately at fast than slow speeds suggests that her *motor coordination is adequate* for the task. If she had difficulty controlling her movement to hit the drum, we would expect her to find it easier at a slower tempo, as she would have more time to make and coordinate the movements. Although people with Down syndrome use different arm movements when they play drums, the effect on accuracy is not significant (Rin-genbach *et al.*, 2006).

Like Chloe, young children also become *less* accurate when tapping or drumming slowly. This is because they need more attention and self-control to drum slowly than quickly, and because the duration between taps is longer at slower speeds. Like motor control, attention and memory span increase with age; young children become better at entraining to slow speeds and these abilities develop. People with Down syndrome and other types of developmental delay can have a *short auditory memory span*. Most adults of Chloe's age can recall sequences of seven to nine numbers (a digit span). Chloe's memory for auditory-verbal information is just two digits, whereas Georgina's digit span is three. The 'phonological loop' in which we temporarily store sounds has a limited capacity (see Figure 2.4). We can liken the loop to a piece of cassette tape that is just long enough for one or two seconds of a recording. At a tempo of 120 bpm, there is half a second between each beat: if Chloe's phonological loop records just under one second of sound, she cannot fit both tap 1 and tap 2 on the tape – so she cannot calculate how long there is between each tap. Whereas Georgina, whose phonological loop might hold one and a half seconds of sound, can record both taps and work out the duration between them. This small difference in auditory memory makes it much harder for Chloe to drum slowly as more memory capacity is needed to store patterns where there is a long time between successive beats.

While hearing and memory are significant factors for Chloe, we also need to examine *experiential* and *physiological* factors. Chloe and Georgina face similar physiological challenges, such as hypotonia, hypermobility and difficulties with motor coordination. However, Georgina has had much more practice than Chloe in playing to the beat. Considerable evidence shows that people with Down syndrome improve motor skills with practice (Sacks & Buckley, 2003), and Georgina's body and brain will have become more efficient at perceiving beat and making and monitoring movements to the beat. Both are likely to have auditory processing disorders, which can slow or degrade the sound signal. However, Chloe's high level of hearing loss can cause more significant difficulties in processing sound and make it harder for her to simultaneously process sound and her own movement. Finally, both have a poor memory for sound, but Chloe's auditory memory span is a digit shorter than Georgina's. This difference is crucial when it comes to 'hearing' patterns in sound and for tracking patterns over time. This affects the ability to drum and has consequences for speech perception.

The following section will explore the links between beat entrainment and speech skills in more detail and review the evidence that developing beat entrainment accuracy can support speech perception in people vulnerable to speech and language differences.

CAN WE USE BEAT ENTRAINMENT TO SUPPORT SPEECH AND LANGUAGE?

The ability to tap to a beat is correlated with a range of speech and language skills, but there is conflicting evidence that teaching someone to tap to a beat will lead to better *language* outcomes. Language is an advanced cognitive skill that takes decades to develop and relies on how other conceptual and cognitive skills develop. However, there is consistent evidence that practice in beat entrainment can have 'near-transfer' effects: activities such as tapping in time may support attention to temporal phenomena and recruit and strengthen some of the same brain regions and pathways that we need for speech perception (Fujii & Wan, 2014; Patel, 2011, 2014). In particular, research with typically developing children has shown that training in rhythm skills can improve *auditory processing skills* (e.g. Kraus & Chandrasekaran, 2010), which is a difficulty common to many learning needs, including *Down syndrome*, *central auditory processing disorder*, *cerebral palsy*, *autism*, *dyslexia*, *hearing loss* and *ADHD*. For children and adults, activities such as playing to a beat can improve how quickly the brain responds to sound, including in children with hearing loss (Hidalgo *et al.*, 2017). Therefore, rhythmic music training has the potential to support and develop the processes that help sound perception in people who have problems perceiving speech sounds.

Such activities might even support language processing and production. Rhythmic training has led to measurable improvements in phonological perception and reading in some children with dyslexia and hearing loss and in children with language delays. Typically, these interventions help children become better at detecting phonemes – the building blocks of words – and can enhance early reading skills (see Gordon, Fehd & McCandliss, 2015, for a review). However, the jump from tapping a beat, to speech, then to language and reading, is considered 'far-transfer'. The evidence for far-transfer of skills is limited, contradictory and contested.

Nevertheless, music training is likely to support the skills that are 'near-transfer' such as listening, attention to sound and tracking of sound. These skills are essential in music and language. Additionally, music may be especially promising for 'children who have language difficulties and therefore much room for improvement' (Swaminathan & Schellenberg, 2020, p.2345). Still, if we are to expect any of these skills to improve and transfer to language, we must understand how to teach beat timing in music and how we can adapt teaching to reduce the effects of perceptual, motoric and sensory limitations. The first step to developing accurate beat perception and production is to use movement, especially movement that engages the whole body.

The importance of movement in beat timing

Moving to music may be crucial in supporting beat perception. As children and as adults, how we move to music can affect how we perceive it. Building on a series of experiments with young children, Phillips-Silver and Trainor (2007) trained young adults to bounce in time with another adult to an 'ambiguous' rhythmic sequence. Half the adults bounced on alternate beats in a rhythmic sequence that gave a sense of 'double time' (such as a march), and half the adults bounced to the patterns that created the sense of 'triple time' (such as a waltz). The participants were subsequently asked to listen to two versions of the original ambiguous track: one new version had been altered to sound more waltz-like and the other more march-like. Participants were asked to identify which pattern was most like the one they had heard previously. All identified as the 'same' the rhythmic pattern that best matched the sequences of movements they made. This was followed by further experiments that tested whether moving was essential or whether seeing another move to the music influenced participants' judgement. The results showed that participants were strongly influenced by their movement experience, as were infants in previous studies. Their studies emphasize that 'sensory perception cannot be separated from the multisensory experience of our bodies' (p.543): in other words, we hear what we feel.

This evidence reinforces the value of movement to build an understanding of musical form. Music approaches such as Dalcroze Eurythmics and Kodály teach students to move in specific ways to 'embody' the music. For example, the student might listen for the 'strong beat' and respond to what they hear by making movements in time that symbolize the pattern. For example, if walking to 4/4 music (four beats in a bar), they may take a heavy step on the first beat of the bar and lighter steps on beats 2, 3 and 4. In 3/4 music (waltz time), they might stomp on beat 1 and trot lightly on beats 2 and 3. The philosophy is that we gain a physical experience and understanding of what we are hearing, and we become practised at listening for sounds and patterns of sound. People trained in these types of music education can use their bodies to express what they hear, internalize the sound, and ultimately learn to represent the sound as musical notation. I have used these approaches to teach adults who have severe learning difficulties to write and read simple musical notation. The section 'Advanced beat-timing skills and games' (at the end of this chapter) will show you how you might begin this process when the child or young adult is ready.

Making movements in time to the beat can influence and fine tune our perception and ability to hear the beat. While we can develop this at any age, movement activities that involve the vestibular system may be critical, especially for children at risk of hearing loss or impairment. The vestibular system is part of the inner ear, and it helps us coordinate balance and get a sense of our orientation. People with hearing loss can have problems with their vestibular system, causing balance and coordination difficulties and poor posture, as was seen in Chloe. We can engage the vestibular system by using movements that cause us to move our heads. Indeed, activities such as dancing and using rhythmic whole-body movements strengthen balance and coordination in deaf children and adults with intellectual disabilities (Fotiadou *et al.*, 2002, 2009). For people at risk of hearing loss and motor coordination difficulties, whole-body rhythmic movements may be essential for developing perception of the beat.

PRACTICAL ACTIVITIES TO SUPPORT BEAT PERCEPTION AND PRODUCTION

Perception in music must be developed before production: production skills typically emerge when a degree of volitional motor control has been achieved. The following activities explain how to make teaching and learning multisensory; they support weaknesses in perception and encourage sensory integration. The activities are based on how typically developing infants and children learn skills to entrain and are presented in developmental order, beginning from birth. I include suggestions for how you could adapt activities for older learners and to meet specific needs. Given that many children and young people can have physical difficulties when moving, please do seek additional guidance from physical therapists to ensure you are working safely.

Early motor and perceptual skills from birth to about 2 years developmental age

SUPPORTING BEAT PERCEPTION

Sing to them. Songs tend to capture the attention more than speech. You can draw attention to the beat in the songs or rhythmic speech by emphasizing the strong beats: most carers do this instinctively.

Help them to feel whole-body movements to the beat. A movement that involves the whole body can help children and young people feel the beat, and support the developing vestibular system. For example, you might put a very young child in a baby bouncer or rocker and gently move them to the strongest pulse of music. As they develop strength in holding their head and upper body, you might hold them on your knee and gently bounce them as you sing a song or listen to music. However, some infants may find movements startling or uncomfortable, especially if they have hearing loss, or difficulties with sensory integration (we will look at this in Chapter 4, especially).

Make it multisensory. Young children and adults with differences in auditory processing or hearing might have difficulty hearing or perceiving the beat. You can provide visual and tactile support to help them become aware of the beat. You could tap in time on their knees or hands, so they can see and feel the pattern. You could use colourful objects or favourite toys and make them 'dance' to music. You could tap on their body so they can feel it – experiment and see what they like! If you have space, a resonance board (easily made from plywood) enables them to lie down and feel the vibrations of the pulse through their body. As they develop an upright posture, encourage them to place their hands on a drum or other resonant instrument or object (a balloon or a bottle might work), and let them feel the vibrations as you tap it. Place their fingers on your throat and sing or say the beat.

SUPPORTING BEAT PRODUCTION

Assist movements to the beat. Most babies will spontaneously move their arms and legs in response to music by about five months – the more salient the beat, the more excitedly they respond. Encourage this movement at very early stages of development, and do it with them. For older learners, subject to their preferences, you could take their hands or feet and move them in time, or put tactile or noisy objects within reach and encourage them to move them. These are good opportunities for you to support developing motor skills too.

Practise moving in time to music. There is plenty of evidence from music therapy that making repetitive movements in time to music can make it easier for children to move and make movements more enjoyable. Remember that most very young children cannot consistently move to a beat, so do not worry about accuracy in production – instead, focus on giving opportunities to move and reinforcing perception and awareness of beats in different types of music.

Emerging skills (about 2–5 years developmental age)
SUPPORTING BEAT PERCEPTION
Support for perception can be reduced as the child develops and the focus can be placed instead on making well-timed movements to the beat. However, older children and adults may need continuing support to 'hear' meter and different levels, or hierarchies, of beat.

Move to music to learn more about meter and beat hierarchies. We can perceive and move to different levels – or hierarchies – of beat in music (Figure 2.2). In part, the way we move or play along to a beat depends on what level we perceive, but it also depends on our preferred motor tempo. Even as adults, it can be difficult to perceive different hierarchies of beat: this is something that may need to be taught. Younger children tend to tap at the fastest rate – the perceived beat that is closest to the music's surface (Kalender, Trehub & Schellenberg, 2013). You may need to model lower beat hierarchies or use different movements – such as large steps for half time (every other beat), and smaller steps to every beat. You could play a game in which you place markers on the floor and you step or jump alternate beats, for example.

Listen to rhythms from many genres and cultures. We can extend and challenge the child's perception of beat by encouraging them to listen to and move to a range of musical styles. For example, you could begin with music that has strong, simple beats, such as most pop or rock music where the first beat is accented; then use music that has a less overt beat so they need to 'find' it. You could introduce music that has more complex metrical structures, such as Indian music that uses over 100 different types of meter (Kalender *et al.*, 2013); these provide an opportunity for counting, as this type of rhythm usually consists of cumulative patterns (e.g. 3+4+3+4). You can also listen to music that has no dominant beat, such as music played by one instrument or voice. The more we can expose ourselves and the child to a range of musical styles and meter, the more we can help them develop their perception of it.

Continue to provide multisensory representations of the beat. Draw attention to different beats and hierarchies through your own movements and by tapping them on the child's shoulder, arms, and so on, or by placing their feet on yours as you move. They might also benefit from visual stimuli to emphasize the beat, such as flashing lights or moving objects. For example, there is an increasing choice of rhythm games available for technology that encourage movements to a beat. Games that provide somatosensory or haptic feedback may be especially helpful – for example, there are wearable metronomes that 'buzz' the beat.

Use props and games to support beat perception. Balls, beanbags, scarves, parachutes and giant scrunchies are all great ways to develop a physical and visual perception of the beat and can form part of musical games. In Dalcroze Eurhythmics, weighted gymnastic balls are used to encourage motor timing to the beat and reinforce a physical sense of the beat. In pairs, a large ball can be bounced between partners in time to music; or the ball can be rolled if this is more appropriate for developing motor skills. It is common in many children's singing games to pass objects in time to the beat – not only can this support beat awareness, but it also supports coordination and timing of motor movements. In pairs or groups, scarves, parachutes and scrunchies provide a visual and physical sense of the beat – standing in a group, an adult or older child can lead a rhythmic movement up and down, thereby encouraging physical awareness of the beat.

SUPPORTING BEAT PRODUCTION

Begin with encouraging motor movements that they already find easier to do. For example, if they have not yet mastered walking or jumping, they will find it very difficult to move independently in time, with accuracy and with safe, controlled movements. In this case, begin with guided activities, in which you make the movements with them – feet on feet, supported bouncing, hand-over-hand tapping, and so on. When they are ready, reduce your physical support and move where they can see you make the movements themselves. Encourage them to play along with you as you tap on drums, pots, pans – whatever you have to hand. Again, when they are ready, encourage the expression of the beat through different movements, from flapping arms to tapping fingers. Their natural tendency is likely to be to make large or fast movements, partly as they will perceive faster beats more easily. However, for those children who have hypermobility or poor proprioception (such as people with Down syndrome, and some people with autism, ADHD, dyspraxia), encourage keeping movements within range. If in doubt, model and ask for smaller movements, with control of speed, rather than large movements that draw on momentum.

Supporting precision in beat timing (about 5–10 years developmental age)

As motor skills and coordination develop, you can use movement activities with props to support the young person's ability to time motor movements to the beat. They can throw and catch balls to slow and fast music, bounce and catch them, and pass them. They can create and perform a series of motor movements, adding a new movement to each beat – so the first beat might be a stamp of the left foot, the second might be a step on the right foot and a clap, and so on. Simple props such as empty drinks bottles or commercially available Boomwhackers can be used to extend their arms and they can use these to hit parts of their body in sequence – thereby getting strong physical and auditory feedback as well as using proprioception skills.

Keep moving. The activities suggested for infants can be continued and developed, and incorporated into a wider range of physical activities, once the child begins to gain greater motor skills. Dancing with them to the music will help them to see and feel the beat. As hearing loss can remain intermittent throughout childhood for some children who experience glue ear, it may also be helpful to continue whole-body exercises that stimulate the vestibular system. Bearing in mind that some young people need additional support for motor activities, you might help them to bounce on a trampoline in time to music and to take part in gross motor movements, such as walking, jumping and skipping to the beat.

Begin to make movements on different levels of the beat. We can encourage the perception of different levels of beat by making movements to different beats, deliberately. For example, by stamping on beat 1 only, and clapping on beat 3; or by playing to the offbeat (beats 2 and 4), which produces a syncopated rhythm, we associate more closely with Jamaican-style music such as Reggae or Ska. This latter can be very tricky as our attention is naturally drawn to the strong first beat!

Practising passing, throwing, bouncing balls to the beat can also encourage accuracy in timing and dexterity. You can use such activities to draw awareness to meter: for example, by making stronger movements on the accented beat.

Advanced beat-timing skills and games

Clap to a metronome. This is something you and your young person can do together to practise accuracy at different tempos. It will help you both learn what sort of tempo suits your learner best – you can find audible metronomes online, or purchase one: some have lights and vibration, too, which can support beat perception.

Develop inner audiation. Develop an inner sense of the beat by asking your child to keep playing on real or 'air' instruments when the music stops. Counting games can also be used to develop inner audiation: challenge your child to play on or move to specific numbers of the beat while saying the beat to metrical patterns of 1234, 123, 123456, 12345678. Decide which numbers to play on or move to and which numbers to keep still on. Set a beat by counting the full sequence first, then play or move only on the numbers. At first, ask them to count along, then gradually reduce the volume to a whisper, then 'think' the numbers. Experiment to find out what they are best at and gradually increase the level of the challenge.

Find the heartbeat of a song. Ask your child to demonstrate the 'heartbeat' of the song – the pulse or beat that goes from the first note until the final note has faded. Sing a simple song that you both know and count how many heartbeats there are in one or two phrases – or the whole song, if they are confident at counting! Explain that we can use a heart symbol to represent the heart and that you can conduct the song by tapping the heartbeats. The same song can be fast or slow but once it has started, it should stay the same speed! Take it in turns to 'conduct' the song, singing and clapping or playing in time to the heartbeat. Watch out for the silent beats (represented by 'z' for 'shhhhh!'): these continue in the song and should be counted and played even though you do not sing on them. There is an example of this activity in Video 5 in the online resources.

CHAPTER SUMMARY

Rhythmic movement and verbal learning are deeply connected; their connections are so strong that an ability to move in time is associated with vocal learning in birds and can predict aspects of language learning in humans. Both skills depend on an ability to perceive very fast changes in sound; to store the duration between sounds; to compare and monitor our own movements to the perceived beat. If we wish to move in time to an auditory beat, we also need to integrate multiple signals from our own body, and we must map these against what we hear. This set of skills can be hard for people who are born with sensory or cognitive differences. They may have to work much harder to perceive or remember the rhythmic template; they may have to work harder to control their own physical movements; they might not easily integrate the complex signals. However, we can support them in developing these skills. In general, we must first ensure that they have opportunities to listen to music, and to see or feel the beat – we might show them the beat, tap it on them, or move them to it. Later, we can focus on helping them move to the beat, using a tempo and type of movement that most suits them; we can make the pulse or meter easier to perceive by using multisensory forms of teaching and feedback; we can continue to adjust our teaching and support until they can make their 'best' timed movement. In doing this, we are helping them train their brain to hear the rapid changes we need for speech perception. At the same time, we are setting up strong foundational skills in music-making.

RECOMMENDED READING

Honing, H. (2019). *The Evolving Animal Orchestra: In Search of What Makes Us Musical*. Cambridge, MA: MIT Press.

Houlahan, M. & Tacka, P. (2015). *Kodály Today: A Cognitive Approach to Elementary Music Education*. Oxford: Oxford University Press.

Kodály Center: The American Folk Song Collection, https://kodaly.hnu.edu.

Patel, A.D. (2008). *Music, Language, and the Brain*. Oxford: Oxford University Press.

Turnbull, F. (2018). *Learning with Music: Games and Activities for the Early Years*. Abingdon, Oxfordshire: Routledge.

CHAPTER 3

Rhythmic Connections – Communication, Music and Verbal Language

THE BIG QUESTIONS

How can we define rhythm in speech, communication and music? How do these skills develop, and why might music support verbal rhythm skills?

By the end of this chapter, you will know:

- which factors influence perception of rhythm in communication, spoken language and music
- milestones in how a typical child develops rhythm skills in communication, speech and music
- why rhythmic training can improve speech in children and young people with developmental speech and language needs.

WHO IS THIS FOR?

The information in this chapter applies to any developing child, and to any child or young person who has verbal differences. It may be of particular interest to those working with children with language or literacy difficulties, such as *dyslexia* or *developmental language disorder*. These are the topics that have been most frequently investigated in rhythm-language research.

This chapter focuses on the connections between rhythm in communication and rhythm in music. I begin by examining the rhythms of early social communication before focusing on what qualities help define and distinguish rhythm in music and speech. Next, I describe how our musical rhythm skills develop in early childhood, and how rhythm, movement and speech are linked as we develop.

This chapter builds on Chapter 2 (pulse). Rhythm depends on the same physical, sensory and cognitive elements we need for beat perception and entrainment, but rhythm demands more of us. This chapter sets the scene for Chapter 4, in which we will explore in greater detail why some children and young people do not easily develop motor rhythms in music or speech; and for Chapter 5, in which we explore practical strategies to support rhythm perception and production in music and speech.

RHYTHM IN COMMUNICATION

In communication – as in the wider world – rhythm exists at different levels and scales. Most of our communicative rhythms have natural variability – far from the machine-like tick of the beat. Rhythm is mutable: to use its Greek etymology, rhythm is *flow*. We find rhythm in the 'large' scale of interpersonal interaction: for example, in the give-and-take of conversation, in the turn-taking and imitation of play, movement or talk, and in the verbal and non-verbal cues we give to show we are listening, or that we understand. At a smaller scale, we hear rhythm in the spoken or sung phrase itself, based on how we 'shape' the phrase and how we emphasize certain words or syllables. At the smaller, increasingly 'fine-grained' levels, spoken rhythm depends on the way we contrast long versus short vowels, and on how long it takes for us to articulate speech sounds.

Rhythms help us make sense of our world and provide a framework for our developing linguistic, cognitive, social and emotional skills. When we are born, we are already tuned into the rhythmic nature of our parental language, but we learn the rhythmic flow of communication in our first months. Face-to-face play, for example 'peek-a-boo', has clearly defined rhythmic properties that can be seen as precursors to language, such as overt stop-start cues, and contrasts of fast/slow, loud/quiet. These types of game help us to anticipate when it is our turn, and encourage us to signal that we want to carry on. In these games, our caregivers might exaggerate the turn-taking cues – they might use sudden changes in volume, extended silence, dramatic gesture or touch to signal that a game is suspended, inviting us to prompt them to continue. Our caregivers encourage us to lead these games, too: they mirror our own infant rhythms when they echo our movements, our babbling and vocal play, so we are leading the interaction:

> A few weeks after birth, a normally developing baby is more alert and able to take part in long protoconversations (Bateson, 1975), drawing family members into intimate rhythmic engagements, making them feel affectionate and causing them to use a special kind of moving and talking that is both dancing and singing.
>
> *(Trevarthen, 2008, p.23)*

Bispham (2006) describes these 'protoconversations' as a 'loose, subconscious use of pulse as a framework' but with deliberate deviations. We use the framework to help the child learn the rules of the game, then we deviate from our rules to encourage interaction and to create an emotional response. For example, we might suddenly stop singing a favourite song, or pause a game mid-flow. This unexpected violation sparks interest and a communicative or emotive response from the child – a look, a laugh, a gesture or word. Through these games, the child begins to learn the rules of conversational turn-taking, and to use voice, looking and movement to maintain and prompt social interaction. At the same time, the games support parental bonding, emotional regulation and the infant's sense of their own physical self – all backed up with praise, smiles, attention and other social reinforcers.

We embody rhythms from an early age, unconsciously echoing the rhythms of others in even small movements. For example, newborns will suck and move their limbs in patterns that echo maternal speech rhythms. This embodiment of rhythm is central to later communication abilities: with careful timing, we use physical movements such as gesture, nodding and eye gaze to maintain emotional and social connection, as well as to indicate our own understanding. As we will see in Chapter 5, we can draw on these principles of early rhythmic learning to support communication and speech in children and young adults who have not yet developed these skills.

WHAT BRAIN AND BODY PROCESSES HELP US PRODUCE RHYTHM?

When we communicate or play with rhythmic timing, our brain is modulating the timing and expression of our limbs and fine motor systems; it is directing and regulating our attention to sensory modalities, including what we hear, see and feel; it is weaving together information from our body and our environment; and it is constantly monitoring and fine tuning what we *do* against what we *plan* to do. Writing about our rhythmic capacity in music, Colwyn Trevarthen, Professor of Psychology and Psychobiology, argues that our musicality – our capacity to be musical – depends on our brain's ability to coordinate *all* of the body's systems as though they were one single system. Through research, Trevarthen identified and located the brain regions that produce these 'body-maps in the brain'. He explained that these regions are 'intricately combined with the neurochemical systems of emotion. The same activating neurons that select movements and control their energy and smoothness also cause changes in the emotions felt, and the intensity and "colour" of consciousness' (Trevarthen, 1999, p.161).

The connection between movement and emotion makes rhythm hard to resist. Most people are drawn towards synchrony, naturally and subconsciously (Gill, 2012). For example, in music, adults tend to spontaneously adapt to the group's tempo, following the dominant beat even as it speeds up or slows down – it takes conscious effort to refuse to go with the flow. We synchronize in our social interactions, too: we tend to move in time with another, use the same gestures, breathe and speak at the same rate, temporarily, at least (e.g. see Mayo & Gordon, 2020). These shared physical and temporal rhythms give us a sense of being in harmony or in tune with another person. However, our rhythmic abilities in communication and music depend on the smooth integration of motor and sensory systems: when our senses are processed and merged seamlessly, our rhythms synchronize, we interact more comfortably and we develop a sense of social connection.

Conversely, when these systems are not operating smoothly – for example, when there is perceived mistiming in our verbal interaction, our gesture or in the integration of sensory information in the brain – we feel discomfort or disconnected. If a parent mistimes their response, an infant will show signs of distress; and an infant or child who is out of sync with their parent or carer can also seem hard to reach (Trevarthen, 2009). For example, Pat Amos (2013) describes why timing is critical for parent-baby interactions at multiple levels, from wake-sleep patterns to bodily movements and vocalizations. Amos writes:

Timing seems to operate as the common link that binds sensory

DEVELOPING EARLY VERBAL SKILLS THROUGH MUSIC

experiences into a coherent whole. Infants move in carefully-timed synchrony with caregivers in a dance-like exchange that creates the framework for a child's first experiences of actors, actions, and things acted on. (Amos, 2013, p.4)

She explains that some parents of infants with autism report that their child's cycles of sleeping, feeding and movement are different from their own. They seem to have different experiences of time, and their rhythms do not always coincide: 'When the timing of these early experiences is "off" it can trigger a cascade of consequences for development' (Amos, 2013, p.4).

Music is a potent agent for supporting communication at multiple levels – neurologically, physically, emotionally and socially – despite the complex factors that can affect our interpersonal rhythms. We will explore this further in Chapter 4.

RHYTHM IN MUSIC, LANGUAGE AND SPEECH

After the physical and acoustic properties of sound itself, rhythm is possibly the most significant property common to music, speech and language. Rhythm is such a powerful part of spoken communication that some cultures can use rhythmic drumming as a substitute for speech. For example, the Bora people of the Amazonian rainforest can use tonal drums to talk. A combination of pitch contrast (high tone versus low tone) and durational contrast emulates the phonemes of their language accurately enough for conversations to take place between groups of people who are 20 km apart. The variation in rhythmic duration as they play allows them to communicate vowel length and some consonants. Incidentally, the maximum difference in time between contrasting rhythm words in the Bora drum language is 20 ms (Seifart *et al.*, 2018). A duration of 20 ms is also the smallest duration we can distinguish in speech or music, and is pretty much as close as we can physically get when matching movements to a beat (see Chapter 2). The connections between music and speech are deep, and pre-conscious, but physiological and perceptual factors constrain them.

Rhythm in music and speech can be described in terms of time, but as we saw in Chapter 2, duration is just one element of rhythm. For example, if a musician plays a rhythmic piece (without pitch), from notation they can read duration (e.g. full notes, quarter notes), tempo (e.g. beats per minute), metrical accent and dynamics. They might then add nuance to these basics, according to their own style and abilities. Rhythm in speech can also be simplified into measures of time (e.g. the relative duration of syllables and speaking (or articulatory) rate), and represented in transcription (e.g. the phonetic alphabet) but this only captures the 'coarse' elements of rhythm, and in a rather abstract form.

The rhythm of speech is notoriously difficult to define, as it is multidimensional. Our perception of speech rhythm is intertwined with pitch (Cumming, 2010) and even if we limit our focus to duration, our ability to perceive syllabic rhythm in single words depends on multiple acoustic cues (e.g. Alexandrou *et al.*, 2016). Furthermore, our rhythm varies according to language, context, individual characteristics and our emotional and physiological state. For example, we might talk more quickly if we are excited or in a rush, more slowly if we are calm, or tired. In conversation, rhythm becomes increasingly hard to quantify, as we must navigate conversational turns, social conventions, and we will use paraverbal rhythmic cues such as gesture and 'fillers' (such as 'er', 'mm', 'uh') to support our meaning and maintain turn and connection with our conversational partner.

It is not possible, in this book, to explore the rhythms of language in depth (please see the recommended reading section at the end of this chapter). Instead, we are concerned with the elements of rhythm that are shared between music and language. In his book *Music, Language, and the Brain*, Patel (2008) defines rhythm as 'the systematic patterning of sound in terms of timing, accent and grouping' (p.96). I will examine each element of his definition in turn, with a view to understanding how they contribute to our sense of rhythm in music and language.

Timing in rhythm

Timing refers to the duration between successive beats, notes or syllables. For music, Patel's definition of rhythm applies both to the *isochronous* and *non-isochronous* rhythm. In most Western music, the pulse is isochronous: each beat, each tap of the hand or foot is equally spaced in time, and this pattern repeats throughout the song, even if the tempo or the meter shifts. Published research examining the relationship between music and language has focused on isochronous rhythm: as we saw in Chapter 2, the ability to perceive changes in energy across time helps us perceive pulse, meter and stressed syllables.

In contrast to isochrony, a *non-isochronous* rhythm in music allows for unequal timing between notes or beats. These non-isochronous patterns are laid over the pulse – these rhythms could be the song's words, drum patterns, a melody line or guitar riffs, for example. This type of rhythm involves change. Unlike the pulse, rhythms do not need to repeat perfectly; and as music therapist Dorita Berger writes, rhythm helps keep us interested and focuses our attention:

> A pattern consists of a variety of rhythmic interjections often teasing about a pulse, organized in such ways as to bring about anticipation and changes of input over a paced beat. Off-beats in jazz are perfect examples of patterns teasing the strictness of pulse. In the broader perspective, rhythm is a perfect integration of pulse plus patterned lengths of sound flowing above, between, against, or parallel to the beat. Pulse must remain steady. Pattern can be freer, erratic, always changing, with stops, starts, fast, slow, combined to add depth and dimension to the constant, faithful pulse. (Berger, 2002, p.116)

There is no guiding pulse in natural, conversational speech. Some forms of language, such as poetry or song, might have a sense of pulse, but in most forms of speech, the relative duration of syllables is the critical factor. Together with tone and pitch, relative duration gives languages a rhythmic 'flavour' that helps us begin to decode speech and discriminate our parental language from other languages (as we will see below). In spoken English, we tend to alternate between long and short vowel durations. This contrast contributes to what we perceive as natural-sounding spoken English. In English, specific rules govern the timing of syllables in most – but not all – words. For example, most two-syllable nouns have a first syllable that has a longer duration than its second syllable; whereas most two-syllable verbs have a longer second syllable:

Nouns: **ba**by, **mu**mmy, **da**ddy, **na**nny, **bi**scuit

Verbs: be**gin**, re**ply**, a**muse**, dis**like**, des**troy**

However, temporal flexibility is necessary for speech. In spoken English, when we combine words into sentences, we might shorten or lengthen some syllables to emphasize certain words and to avoid having too many stressed syllables occurring together; we use a process of 'vowel reduction' to help maintain a clear pattern of long-vs-short. In music, we tolerate very little variability in timing: if someone's duration between beats is more than 5 per cent off the target, we will notice it! But in speech, we can tolerate more variation (33%) before unusual timing affects our understanding (Patel, 2008).

Although durational cues help us track and understand speech and music, relative duration is just one factor. Durational changes work alongside the other aspects of rhythm (accent, and grouping, below) to help provide rhythmic patterning in speech and music.

Accent in rhythm

Accent refers to the way that some sounds in music and speech are more salient than others: this saliency is driven by subtle changes of timbre and pitch, as well as by changes in duration. The duration *between* accented syllables is an important factor in giving spoken language its rhythmic flavour: in spoken English, these peaks tend to occur every 300–500 ms, which broadly corresponds to our preferred range of tempos for music. Just as accent contributes to our sense of rhythm in spoken English, metrical accent gives music its sense of movement. As discussed in Chapter 2, in most Western music, subtle changes in sound mark the 'strong' beats of the bar, which is usually the first beat. This gives the music a characteristic we can hear and feel – a 2/2 or 4/4 is something we might march to, a 3/4 meter is something we might waltz to, and a 6/8 lends itself to skipping (see Chapter 2, Figure 2.2).

Grouping in rhythm

In music and speech, we perceive clusters of notes or words that seem to belong together. In language, these groups create meaningful units, such as short phrases or whole sentences. In music, we perceive these as rhythmic patterns, motifs, riffs. Our perception of grouping in each domain depends on multiple acoustic factors, including those related to timing and accent – but additional cues help us perceive the boundaries. There might be silence before or after each phrase – this helps us to easily perceive separate blocks of sound. However, we also rely on more subtle cues: towards the end of a phrase in music or speech we might notice a lowering of pitch and volume, a lengthening of duration, and subtle changes in timbre (see Videos 1 and 2 in the online resources for an example).

WHAT FACTORS AFFECT OUR RHYTHM
FOR SPEECH AND MUSIC?

In music and language, our rhythmic skills depend on how we track and process changes in duration, stress and grouping. As we have seen, these skills might develop differently in some people, according to their perception of sound (Chapter 1), and developmental and cognitive factors (e.g. Chapter 2). We need to perceive rhythm before we can produce it; and production demands a lot of our brain and body in terms of cognition and movement. In Chapter 2, we looked at how the brain planned a simple temporal sequence (the pulse), but if we wish to play, speak or sing with *expressive* rhythmic timing (duration + accent + grouping), the motor centres of our brain must formulate a complex motor plan. This plan instructs our relevant muscles (limbs, vocal muscles, oro-motor muscles) to move, and lets them know when and in what sequence to move, for how long and how quickly. High degrees of speed and motor coordination are needed for speech – in a fluent language, most people produce 15 speech sounds a second, or approximately four to seven syllables a second. The accuracy of our speech depends on how well we can coordinate motor movements in our speech articulators – such as our tongue, lips, soft palate – and our voice. As such, we are constrained by neuromuscular, anatomical and respiratory abilities as well as by cognitive abilities (we will examine these in later chapters). Our brains also plan the subtle motor adjustments that alter our speaking pitch, volume and timbre. This is a pre-conscious act that takes milliseconds (5–20 ms, Trevarthen, 1999). Unsurprisingly, we often make mistakes when executing these motor plans. This can lead to speech 'errors' such as mistimings, misarticulations and spoonerisms – such as, 'The Lord is a shoving leopard', which is an error attributed to William Archibald Spooner, minister and Oxford don, who intended to say, 'The Lord is a loving shepherd'.

Just as speech depends on the combined movement of our articulators, voice and breath, no instrument can produce a rhythmic sound without some movement and force being applied to it. Even an instrument like a Soundbeam, that is tailored to respond to the smallest movement such as blinking, requires repeated controlled movement to produce a sound that is rhythmic. Playing or saying something rhythmic at speed and with precision and dynamics requires fine motor timing and control. For example, Rimsky-Korsakov's *Flight of the Bumblebee* when played at 144 beats per minute requires about 6.5 finger movements per seconds of the right hand; the 2020 World Record holder plays 810 notes in 50 seconds on a piano, an average speed of 16 movements per second.

Playing or saying a rhythm requires considerable control and awareness of physical movement, in addition to a host of attentional and cognitive factors. As Bispham (2006) puts it, 'musical rhythmic behavior (MRB)' is:

> a constellation of concurrently operating, hierarchically organized, subskills including general timing abilities, smooth and ballistic movement (periodic and nonperiodic), the perception of pulse, a coupling of action and perception, and error correction mechanisms.'

These complex motor, perceptual and cognitive skills take years to develop, as the body and brain mature. Below, I outline the major milestones in rhythm development in music and how these developing skills are related to speech perception and early speech production.

RHYTHMIC DEVELOPMENT
The early years

In Chapter 1, we imagined the way that a developing baby might hear the rhythms of music and language, such as their mother's heartbeat, the sound of her speaking and singing. The evidence of such *in-utero* learning comes from observing how foetuses and newborns respond to language and music. Researchers use changes in heart rate and movement as indicators of attention. For example, newborns show that they recognize songs that they heard in the womb by turning their head towards the sound. Through observational experiments, researchers have learned that most newborns are sensitive to changes in rhythm and tempo in music, and that they can tell apart families of language, based on the languages they heard while in the womb. For example, a child from an English-speaking culture will respond to English or to a language such as Dutch that shares rhythmic characteristics, but they will not show recognition of a language type that has a different type of rhythm (such as Japanese or French) unless they were regularly exposed to it *in-utero* (Mehler *et al.*, 1988; Nazzi, Bertoncini & Mehler, 1998; Gasparini *et al.*, 2021). Furthermore, they can apply these skills to music: from a very early age, infants can segment melody lines into rhythmic units, a skill that supports developing language.

Having already learned a little about its parental language before it is born, the newborn can use rhythm to gradually separate the sound stream into meaningful units of sound. For children of English speakers, the regularity of stressed syllables, and the common pattern of stress versus unstressed syllables, can help them anticipate *when* a strongly accented sound will occur; additional cues such as lengthening at the end of phrases, and pitch changes, will further help them perceive boundaries and to divide what they hear into phrases, groups and syllables. These cues help them focus on the fine-grained changes in sound, too, and to learn which speech sounds are essential for their language. During their first six months in the physical world, the newborn learns which sounds are important and which are not: those sounds that are not heard frequently within early development are deemed culturally irrelevant, and the infant brain learns to stop paying attention to them. For example, the newborn can perceive the speech sounds of all languages, but after about six months, they lose the ability to 'hear' those sounds that do not frequently occur. Between the ages of six and twelve months, infants also lose sensitivity to non-native tones and rhythms, which parallels their reduced ability to discriminate non-native speech sounds. This loss helps infants focus on the sounds that are meaningful within their environment. It also explains why we, as adults, have difficulty discriminating between consonant sounds or pitch changes in unfamiliar languages, and why we can find music of different cultures hard to grasp. Unless we were exposed to the sound early, we do not easily hear the subtle changes in timbre or tone that can differentiate speech sounds, or tune into the different forms of rhythm, pitch and timbre (for more, see Ferguson & Farwell, 1975; Aitchison, 2012).

From birth, songs and song-like speech provide additional scaffolding for learning speech sounds and musical elements. The exaggerated melodies of infant-directed speech, songs and nursery rhymes appeal to the infant's ear. Infant-directed songs and infant-directed speech are slower than adult speech, and the sounds and rhythms are exaggerated. These characteristics can help the newborn perceive patterns in the verbal sound stream and, gradually, to perceive the different rhythmic 'levels' that help us communicate – syllables, words, phrases and turn-taking cues. This style of communication is believed to be universal but the specific acoustic features that a caregiver exaggerates are linked to their culture and language (e.g. Broesch & Bryant, 2015). There is also evidence that the rhythm of a nation's language can influence its non-vocal music

(Patel, 2003). Patel and colleagues investigated this by comparing the rhythms of French and English music to the spoken languages. Research has since shown that the same linguistic rhythms that can distinguish spoken English from French are found in children's songs (Hannon *et al.*, 2016). This early enculturation may help children attune to both their native language and to their wider musical environment.

Development of rhythmic expression

By about four months, an infant can recognize the features of their own name and link frequently heard words, such as 'mummy' and 'daddy' with their caregivers. It may be another six months, though, before they can reproduce what they perceive. Volitional rhythmic production in body movements and speech lag behind perception: skills in rhythmic movement emerge as perceptual and motor systems mature, and as the baby grows physically. Early movements and early sounds are reflexive, rather than intentional: that is, the newborn may startle in response to loud sounds and will cry in response to distress. The newborn produces motor rhythms that are internally driven, such as the rhythm of sucking, or the rhythm of breathing. As the infant develops, they begin to make deliberate movements and vocal responses, supported by a developing neuromuscular system and by social interactions. From two months of age, the infant can adapt the tempo of rhythmic sucking to an external tempo. During these same months, they experiment with musical building blocks of language: coos and gurgles, dramatic vocal glides and swoops, and percussive rhythms of consonants. They play with pitch and timbre in sound, as well as duration: skills that help them learn to differentiate and produce discrete speech sounds and the subtle markers of accent.

By about five months, as their oral musculature develops, the infant can produce long babbling sequences of syllables for their own amusement, or as part of an interactive game with their caregivers. At the same time as the infant begins experimenting with the complex motor movements needed for producing speech, their nervous system has developed control of limb movements. From five to six months, infants begin to respond physically to the rhythm of music, rhythmically banging their hands or kicking their feet. They also increase the pace of their movements in response to increased tempo, although they do not synchronize at this stage. Although they do this in response to motherese, they respond more rhythmically to music, indicating their enjoyment and a preference for highly rhythmic and melodic sound.

At these early stages, research suggests that providing opportunities to explore sound is more important to musical development than providing structured learning.

The school years

Rhythmic speech skills develop rapidly after the first year, as fine oro-motor skills develop. From about three years of age, most children have begun to deconstruct familiar words into their syllables and sounds. Most children can produce the repertoire of native English speech sounds by 5 years, and can control the rhythm of syllables and pitch well enough to place emphatic stress on syllables and produce melodic contours.

As with early speech development, rhythmic motor production skills depend on increasingly refined motor movements and cognitive development. As explained in Chapter 2, rhythm development in the early years is focused mainly on developing accurate timing to the beat. As the infant matures, the early responses to music become more purposeful and controlled, so that between the ages of two and five years, children begin to imitate rhythms vocally and through motor movements. As they become more conscious of their own movements and those of others, they begin to use sensory feedback to alter and refine their productions, gradually becoming more accurate and in time with the sounds they hear. However, motor skills do not develop across all limbs simultaneously; as a result, some types of movement are more suitable for performing rhythms at different ages or stages of development. For example, at three to four years, infants may be most accurate at using oral motor skills to repeat rhythms; accuracy in clapping rhythms does not typically emerge until four to five years. Accuracy in motor timing also depends on maturing cognitive skills. Indeed, the link between developing motor skills and cognitive skills is so strong in the early years that musical ability may be a reliable indicator of non-verbal mental age (MA). Matsuyama (2005) researched rhythmic clapping and melodic skills of 92 Japanese children aged between 6 months and 69 months. His results showed that the ability to clap back rhythms correlated with MA scores at a statistically significant level.

By about five years, most children can tap steadily to a beat but the ability to mark metrical stress takes longer to develop. In a study of 120 pupils aged between five and eight years, most eight-year-olds (83%) could perceive metrical accents but only 50 per cent of the older children could reproduce metrical accents (Drake, Jones & Baruch, 2000). Their rhythmic abilities depended on both motor maturation and attentional skills. Younger children were less able to simultaneously attend to rhythmic form *and* dynamics. In an earlier study, Drake and Gérard (1989) found no difference in the ability to produce metrical rhythms between seven-year-olds and adults. This indicates that rhythmic ability is almost fully developed by seven years. However, some aspects of rhythm continue to develop beyond seven years: for example, some studies report that the ability to play with a metrical accent does not develop until about nine years; beat entrainment develops early, but the ability to entrain to another's rhythm is not developed until about ten years of age, and complex rhythm patterns may take a lifetime to master.

Several studies illustrate that the mode of instruction and production affects performance while motor and attentional skills are developing, and into adulthood. For example, at five years, rhythms based on word syllables are more easily produced than tapped rhythms; rhythms are more easily produced if they are accompanied by sung words, and rhythms are reproduced more easily when they are tapped, rather than presented as part of a melody. In their study of children aged between six and eight years, Schleuter and Schleuter (1989) reported that younger children are better able to perform rhythms when chanting on a neutral syllable ('loo') than by clapping or stepping. Musical education systems such as Kodály and Suzuki stress the need to feel rhythms, as well as to see and hear them. Moving in time to meter is known to shape how infants perceive ambiguous music: being bounced to every other beat primed them to listen for longer to music that was in duple time; being bounced every three beats primed them for music in triple time. Using movements helps to internalize the rhythm – it creates a physical sensation that accompanies the auditory sensation and involves the vestibular system and proprioception, which are closely linked to the auditory system (see Chapter 2, Figure 2.4). Indeed, hearing music can activate the motor areas of the brain, as though the listener were themselves playing. It is therefore important to support a child's experience of rhythm in as many sensory modalities as possible, while being careful not to overwhelm the child with *multiple* simultaneous demands. You may need to experiment to learn which combinations work best for individuals (e.g. auditory + kinaesthetic; auditory + visual: see Appendix 2 in the online resources for example activities).

Section summary

The fastest speed at which we can produce sounds that are both clearly articulated *and* rhythmic depends on a combination of factors, including how much fine motor control we have of the articulators (tongue, lips, jaw); the phonological complexity of sounds and sound combinations; our speaking rate; the familiarity of sounds and words; and our ability to plan motor movements for the whole sentence or phrase. Motor control for speech takes years of practice; even in our first language, it might take ten years before we can speak fluently at speed, without loss of intelligibility. Unusual, novel or complex words or syllables place greater demands on our articulators and involve cognitive processes such as attention and executive control. Until we have mastered the motor patterns for words, our attempts to say them with accurate timing may vary at the phonological level and syllabic level. When it comes to considering the rhythmic skills of people with developmental differences, we must consider their physical capacity as well as perceptual ability, social and cognitive development. Speed and skill can be developed, but there are limits to both that are in part determined by maturational age.

WHY MIGHT MUSIC-BASED RHYTHM SUPPORT SPEECH?

As we saw in the Introduction, extensive music training can lead to improvements in real-world skills, such as better reproduction of rhythmic speech in a second language. For non-musicians, there are also correlations between the speed of rhythmic processing for speech and musical rhythmic abilities. The evidence suggests that those people who have strong rhythmic skills in music have brains that are better able to process rhythm in speech, and those with weaker musical rhythmic skills have poorer abilities to process speech sounds and rhythms. Research is beginning to show that developing rhythmic abilities for music can cause some of these changes at both the neurological level and in terms of functional skills. The most convincing results come from intervention studies that use a test group and a control group. For example, a study by François *et al.* (2013) examined brain responses and speech-related skills in eight-year-olds over a period of two years; half received training in art, and half in music. The use of art as a control measure helped ensure that any positive changes in the music group were not simply the result of taking part in a new or stimulating activity. Participants in each group were matched for age, sex, cognitive ability and socio-economic status. Their results showed that music training led to better abilities in identifying pseudowords from a speech stream of nonsense syllables, as well as faster neural responses to sound. Similar studies have shown that music training can cause changes in speech for adolescents. For example, a group of 14-year-olds took part in either four years of community music or four years of army skills training. The music training led to better phonological skills than the army skills training. These studies provide convincing evidence that music training develops skills in rhythm perception and that these skills benefit speech perception.

The links between rhythmic abilities in music and in language are so strong that poor rhythmic timing may be a risk factor for speech and language disorders. However, rhythmic training can reduce some of this risk. Training in rhythm can support speech processing and production in children with *hearing loss* and in children whose main or only difficulty is learning speech or language, including *developmental language disorder*, *developmental apraxia of speech*, *stuttering* and *dyslexia*. For some of these children, training in music can lead to improved perception of speech, and even to improved grammatical comprehension.

There is a lack of research with children and young people who have more complex learning needs; however, one early study examined rhythm and speech in children with moderate learning disabilities. The children were asked to imitate the clapped syllabic pattern of words before speaking and while speaking. The children were able to speak words with greater rhythmic accuracy after clapping the word rhythms (Jackson, Treharne & Boucher, 1997). More recently, Auditory-Motor Mapping Training (AMMT) has been shown to support children with autism who are non-verbal, and those with emerging verbal skills. AMMT combines rhythmic motor movements (such as drumming) with verbal intonation. The therapy was used with 40 children with autism who did have intelligible speech and used vocal communication rarely. The therapists delivered individual sessions five times a week over an eight-week period. All children used verbal communication more frequently at the end of the intervention and were better able to articulate words and phrases (Wan *et al.*, 2011). Such rhythmic 'priming' is also a key element of Melodic Intonation Therapy (MIT). MIT was designed to help people recover language following trauma to their left hemisphere, such as a stroke. The therapy uses exaggerated forms of prosody of speech to help the brain recover. In one form of MIT, the therapist might half-sing a question, using a limited set of contrasting pitches (high/low) while tapping its rhythm on the patient's left hand. There are strict protocols for MIT, and its success depends on the cause of the language loss. However, some therapists argue that the sensory experience of rhythm – such as the therapist tapping the rhythm on the left hand – is key in priming the brain for speech production (Wan & Schlaug, 2013; Schlaug, Marchina & Norton, 2008). Indeed, the durational component of rhythm in MIT may cause beneficial changes even without the melodic component (Fujii & Wan, 2014); this type of simplified approach may help reduce the complexity of the auditory signal and aid processing for speech.

Recent research shows how different temporal levels of rhythm can support the brain's ability to process speech and language (e.g. see Goswami, 2019a, 2019b). As discussed earlier, we use stress cues to help us identify metrical accent and stress in speech. There are some indications that people with developmental language disorder and dyslexia have difficulties detecting the acoustic cues that distinguish temporal levels of phrase, syllable and sound (Goswami, 2011, 2019a, 2019b; Cumming *et al.*, 2015); and in music, they have difficulties with perceiving meter, as well as with isochronous beats (Chapter 2). However, individuals might have greater difficulties perceiving one level than another. For example, research by Leong and Goswami (2014) indicates that children with *developmental language disorder* may form sub-groups: one group has greater difficulty detecting cues that mark stressed syllables, while the other sub-group has greater difficulty detecting phrase-level cues. In comparison, children with *dyslexia* seem to have difficulty detecting syllables stress and metrical accent. These subtle differences in perception have implications for therapy and teaching. Some children or young people might benefit more from musical tasks that prime the rhythm of the whole phrase than they do from beat entrainment tasks; whereas others with weak phonological skills might benefit more from clapping or marching to word syllables, in time to music (Leong & Goswami, 2014; Cumming *et al.*, 2015). In practice, we might want to work on multiple levels of rhythm perception and production, unless we are delivering targeted one-to-one therapy, with awareness of which level of perception is most affected.

Introducing PRISM theory

The growing body of evidence shows that training in rhythm, especially, can support development of verbal skills. The research evidence has recently led to a framework to explain why rhythm, rather than music in general, might work to support speech skills in groups with developmental speech and language disorders. After reviewing evidence from different disciplines, including music therapy and neuroscience, researchers have proposed that three 'mechanisms' are needed to support rhythmic timing in speech and in music (Fiveash *et al.*, 2021). They argue that 'targeted training of these mechanisms should enhance related skills in both music and speech/language processing'. The mechanisms are:

1. precise, fine-grained auditory processing
2. synchronization/entrainment of neural oscillations to external rhythmic stimuli
3. sensorimotor coupling mechanisms (Fiveash *et al.*, 2021).

As explored in Chapter 2 and above, rhythmic timing in music encourages 'fine-grained auditory processing' (mechanism 1): that is, in music we must attend to temporal changes at different levels, and these levels correspond to the same changes we need to discriminate speech sounds, syllables and rhythm in phrases. As we have seen, music training that involves attention to timing can cause these changes in auditory processing.

We have not yet discussed the idea of entraining 'neural oscillations' (mechanism 2). Neural oscillation is a term that describes how neurons from different areas of the brain, spinal cord and autonomic nervous system synchronize when they are activated. When neurons are activated by a stimulus, they 'oscillate' between a state of 'excitation' and 'inhibition', in a similar way that air particles are activated by movement in air (Chapter 1, Figure 1.1). When we hear a rhythm, activated neurons entrain to the rhythm and echo the rhythmic structure of the stimulus (Zoefel, Ten Oever & Sack, 2018). This process is believed to underlie our abilities to track rhythm (Large, Herrera & Velasco, 2015) and speech (e.g Kösem *et al.*, 2018). It is also linked to attention and helps the communication of rhythm between auditory and motor parts of the brain (Assaneo & Poeppel, 2018). As such, neural entrainment helps us to predict events in time and to track different levels of rhythm in music and in speech (such as meter, hierarchy of the beat, rhythmic pattern, phrase, word, syllable, sound in speech). According to the PRISM theory, if we actively track a specific layer in the rhythm in music, we are using and enhancing the same processes we need for tracking speech.

Mechanism 3 has already been explored in this chapter and in

Chapter 2: if we intend to produce rhythms in music or speech, the connections between auditory and motor systems need to communicate efficiently. Incredibly, just listening to musical or spoken rhythms can ready the motor cortices (see Novembre & Keller, 2014 for a review) but, as we have explored, moving to the rhythm enhances this connection. This framework provides clarity about what we need to put in place in music if we wish to support speech skills in children and young people who have verbal difficulties. The authors of PRISM go on to explain how different types of activity may be useful in supporting different skills: for example, that attention to timing may support the 'fine' processing skills needed for literacy, whereas attention to larger rhythms (such as rhythmic patterns) may support people with speech production skills.

It seems likely that music activities will support speech *perception* because the skills we need to perceive changes in music rhythm are very close to the skills we use for perceiving speech rhythm, and because the skills share networks and processes within the brain. However, the picture is more complex if we extend the same principle to speech *production*. Speech production depends on a more widely dispersed set of skills and neurological processes. Therefore, the cause of speech difficulties is diverse. For example, a speech difficulty may stem from deficits in neurological timing (controlling movement) or motor programming (making movements), from problems with sensory integration, sensory feedback, or from weak muscle tone or reduced motor control. Furthermore, cognitive processes can interfere with speech production. In people who stutter, for example, spontaneous speech is more likely to produce stuttering than repeating an utterance, because spontaneous speech requires our brains to plan for meaning, grammar, rhythm, stress and intonation. (We will return to these discussions in Chapter 9, when we consider songs and singing for speech.) However, when we consider speech production, a focus on producing clear contrasts in the relative duration of syllables in speech *can* make the difference between speech that is intelligible and speech that is not. Speaking with appropriate durational contrasts can support intelligible speech, especially when other cues (such as prosody or articulation) are poor (Nooteboom, 1997). Attention to timing is therefore the first level to support when using music for speech.

CHAPTER SUMMARY

Rhythm helps us to communicate at different levels. It helps us synchronize with others, develop and maintain social connections, and attend to and perceive events around us. In communication, rhythm helps us anticipate events, such as turn-taking, and perceive large and small structures of language, such as phrase boundaries, words, syllables and phonemes.

Our perception of rhythm in music and in speech relies on changes that occur in the acoustic signal, in terms of duration, pitch, intensity and timbre. These cues help accentuate some sounds, beats or syllables. We use these stressed sounds as markers – they can signal patterns (e.g. meter), groups (e.g. phrase) and syllables. Our ability to perceive rhythm in music and speech depends on our perceptual abilities, and these depend on our cognitive and sensory systems, on our physical experiences of rhythm and on enculturation. We rely on these systems in making music, too, but these must be integrated with our motor control, which develops as our bodies and brains mature. Accuracy in rhythmic production for speech depends primarily on our very fine motor skills for articulation, coupled with our ability to control relative duration and timing. Once we have mastered these fine motor skills, we need to learn to adapt the rhythms of words and make additional adjustments to stress patterns so that our speech fits with the conventions of rhythmic stress patterns in spoken English and we can communicate our meaning. Despite the complex issues that affect rhythm for music and speech, we can use rhythmic musical activities to support perception of speech by directing attention to different rhythmic levels. We can use the durational patterns of words and phrases to support perception of speech: this in turn can support intelligible speech production, even when finer motor control is less well developed (e.g. for pitch, intensity, timbre, voice).

RECOMMENDED READING

Aitchison, J. (2012). *Words in the Mind: An Introduction to the Mental Lexicon*. Hoboken, NJ: John Wiley & Sons.

Berger, D.S. (2002). *Music Therapy, Sensory Integration and the Autistic Child*. London: Jessica Kingsley Publishers.

Ferguson, C.A. & Farwell, C.B. (1975). Words and sounds in early language acquisition. *Language*, 51(2), 419–439.

McPherson, G. (ed.) (2015). *The Child as Musician: A Handbook of Musical Development*. Oxford: Oxford University Press.

Stackhouse, J. & Wells, B. (1997). *Children's Speech and Literacy Difficulties: A Psycholinguistic Framework*. London: Whurr.

CHAPTER 4

Understanding Rhythm Difficulties in Communication, Speech and Music

THE BIG QUESTIONS

What types of differences and difficulties do some learners have with rhythmic communication and speech, and why? How do their abilities or difficulties in speech and communication relate to their rhythmic abilities in music? How can rhythmic music make a difference to communication?

By the end of this chapter you will:

- understand the ways that sensory differences can affect social rhythms and (ultimately) verbal communication
- know how rhythmic perception and production can appear in people with:
  - social/communication difficulties (e.g. autism/ADHD)
  - motor-based difficulties (e.g. stuttering, cluttering)
  - complex speech and perceptual differences (e.g. Down syndrome).

WHO IS THIS FOR?

This chapter explores rhythmic timing in learners who have social, sensory and perceptual difficulties, including people with *autism* and *ADHD*. The second section will focus on rhythmic disorders that arise mainly from a motor difficulty, including *stuttering*, *cluttering* and *dyspraxia*. The information is pertinent for those working with people with *Down syndrome* and it has relevance to those with similar motor-based *cerebral palsy difficulties* in *verbal memory, hearing difficulties, hypermobility* and *muscle weakness.*

This chapter focuses on why some children and adults have difficulties perceiving and producing music and speech rhythms. It is split into two sections. The first focuses on how social and sensory differences affect timing. These differences are often reported in learners with autism and ADHD, dyslexia, specific learning difficulties and developmental language disorder. This section discusses how differences in speech fluency, sensory processing and sensory integration can all interrupt the smooth flow of social rhythms. It also explores attentional differences in the context of autism and ADHD. The first section concludes with a summary of the evidence that rhythmic music activities can help develop these skills.

The second section focuses on rhythmic differences that arise primarily from a motor-based difficulty: this includes a discussion of fluency disorders (stuttering, cluttering), motor weakness (dysarthria) and motor timing difficulties (dyspraxia). Many children and young adults have needs that fall into these areas. This section focuses on Down syndrome to show how rhythm might develop differently in motor-music skills, speech production and perception. It explains how rhythm in music can support these skills, despite their complex needs.

SECTION 1: WHY DO SOME CHILDREN AND YOUNG PEOPLE HAVE DIFFICULTIES WITH RHYTHM IN MUSIC AND SPEECH?
Social, sensory and attentional differences

Rhythm is key to building and sustaining relationships, as we saw in Chapter 3. Social rhythms include turn-taking, gesture, posture, breathing, facial expression, eye gaze, voice quality, speech rate and intonation. Each rhythm contributes to social connection, and we can lose this connection when these rhythms are upset. For example, when we communicate with ease, each partner unconsciously adapts their verbal communication to match their conversational partner. When we cannot attune to another's rhythm, we are effectively locked out of communication.

Social rhythms can be affected in people who have *speech fluency disorders* and difficulties with *verbal and non-verbal social cues.* Fluency disorders (*stuttering* and *cluttering*) can lead to disordered, unpredictable timing in speech, which negatively affects the communicative relationship (Borrie, Lubold & Pon-Barrie, 2015). In verbal and non-verbal communication, timing is critical for social interaction. Anticipating *timing* can be problematic for any child or young adult who has difficulties with attention, processing or language. People with *developmental delays* or *altered sensory processing* can experience problems attending to, perceiving or processing paraverbal cues – such as vocal turn-taking signals – or non-verbal cues – such as gesture or eye gaze. These issues can affect rhythmic communication at a 'large' temporal scale. For example, when we talk with a friend and signal that we have finished our 'turn', we expect a response from them within about 250 ms. The listener must be alert to the paraverbal cues that show we intend to finish speaking (e.g. a rising intonation that signals a question or a downward intonation that signals the end of their turn) and they must then be ready to respond, having taken time to process what we have said, interjecting neither too early (interrupting us) nor too late, which risks us speaking again. Attention to multiple cues is needed for rhythmic interaction. This can be incredibly challenging if someone has overlapping sensory differences or problems with attention or self-regulation. We will return to these issues later in this chapter.

We also use rhythmic *entrainment* to support communicative relationships. For example, we subconsciously match gestures or body positions with another, match speaking rates or share joint attention (see Chapter 3). Entrainment has been linked to social and emotional differences in children with autism. For example, a child with autism might experience difficulties in entraining to the subtle cues of others, such as blinking (Nakano, Kato & Kitazawa, 2011) as well as to the more prominent rhythmic cues, such as turn-taking. These skills are usually present in adults with autism, leading some researchers to propose that younger children with autism have delayed development of skills required for speech-based social entrainment (Wynn, Borrie & Sellers, 2018). However, adults might have developed strategies to camouflage aspects of their identity in order to fit in and avoid stigma (e.g. Pearson & Rose, 2021; Miller, Rees & Pearson, 2021). Such masking can damage emotional wellbeing, so we must think carefully whether developing such skills is genuinely helpful to the child or young person.

For some children and young people, rhythmic entrainment skills allow them to participate in and enjoy musical activities with others. We can teach these rhythmic skills using approaches that echo early rhythmic communication. The case study of Nicola, below, shows how the turn-taking structure of singing games helped her to form new relationships with staff and join in with peers.

Case study: Nicola

Nicola is a nine-year-old child with autism and global developmental delay. She rarely talks, preferring to use touch, gesture and PECS (Picture Exchange Communication System) when initiating or responding to others. She is hypersensitive to sound, so music and busy environments can be distressing. As a result, Nicola wears headphones to help reduce the effects of the noise around her.

Nicola took part in six weeks of music-making with other children from her school and another school. During the first session, she seemed unsettled and anxious. As she became used to the new routine and new people, Nicola became more settled and engaged in a broader range of activities. She showed interest in musical activities and games that used puppets and incorporated clear visual, gestural and vocal turn-taking cues. In her third week, Nicola anticipated her turn in some of these songs and began to respond with a look, gesture or touch. In the fourth week, she used her voice for the first time: she whispered 'thank you' in the hello song, greeted the puppet, vocalized during some songs, and named pictures/cards in songs in the appropriate place. As she became more familiar with staff leading the music session, she actively sought interaction with them, using non-verbal communication at first. She was able to initiate some familiar songs and activities through this. According to staff who knew her well, Nicola made excellent progress in turn-taking and anticipatory skills. Staff indicated that it was new for Nicola to want to be involved in group activities.

Connecting through rhythms

We can use physical motor rhythms to develop a social relationship; from there, we can help children and adults who are usually non-verbal to find meaning and enjoyment in verbal communication. One example of a rhythm-based communicative intervention is Intensive Interaction (Nind & Hewett, 1994). Practitioners of Intensive Interaction work with the subtle cues that most of us subconsciously use when we synchronize with another; they look for these cues and make them overt. For example, a practitioner may observe the breathing pattern of a child or adult and imitate the rhythm of their breathing and its rate, intensity and sound. They might use this pattern to create a turn-taking rhythm, emphasizing the breathing movement or sound in short bursts, playing with it and adjusting it in the same way a carer emulates an infant's vocal babbling or coos. The deliberate use of the young person's activity or sound catches their attention and signals a common language. As the practitioner and young person take turns to notice and copy the signal of the other, this rhythmic to-ing and fro-ing creates a communicative bridge, the first step in building a trusting relationship. From this starting point, the young person may begin to communicate with intent – they may use their sound or movement to prompt a turn from the practitioner or may start to echo the breathing or gesture of the practitioner. This rhythmic play is a building block for later verbal communication. With practice, the individual may begin to perceive and attune to a broader range of communicative stimuli as they also develop a rhythmic, non-verbal language with the practitioner.

This approach can support social behaviours such as eye gaze and joint attention and stimulate interest in people and their vocalization. The process works well in a musical context, using voice or instrumental sounds (e.g. Corke, 2014, see Chapter 8). However, the human voice can stimulate vocal production with astonishing effect. In the extract below, Phoebe Caldwell, an experienced Intensive Interaction practitioner who works with people with autism, describes how she uses the sounds made by Pranve, a young adult with autism, to initiate communication. Pranve is hypersensitive to sound, but he responds positively to how Phoebe improvises with the sounds he already makes.

Since Pranve is easily disturbed, when I arrive, I take care not to invade his personal space before making contact with him. So when his mother opens the door I listen – and from another room hear, 'er-er-er', so I respond, 'er-er, er-er-er?', with a lift at the end, rather in the way one might say, 'Hello, how are you?' He comes straight out and takes my hand and leads me to the sitting room. I ask him if I may sit down and he responds by pointing to the chair, so I know he understands at least simple speech.

I sit beside him and respond to each of his small sounds, tuning into how they make me feel, but altering the rhythm or pitch occasionally. I am answering rather than copying. At first he is half turned away from me but he gives me his hand which I shake in time to the sounds we are exchanging. He becomes more interested and turns round to face me, laughing. He introduces new sounds and movements to which I respond. We are soon engaged in a complex non-verbal interactive conversation.

I draw the shape of his different sounds on his forearm and he leans forward and looks with interest, then tries a different sound to which I respond with a shape that reflects its rhythm and pitch. (Caldwell, 2006, p.71)

Phoebe goes on to explain how Pranve begins to engage in singing for the first time; and how his interest in these new forms of communication reduces the effects of his hypersensitivity to environmental noises. Phoebe's description of how Pranve focuses on her vocal patterns, and their visual and tactile counterparts, highlights how focusing on something enjoyable may help reduce someone's sensitivity to sound. Recent studies indicate that children with autism process *more* sound from their environment – rather than being unable to focus on one sound or filter out background sounds, they are more aware of the entire sound spectrum than peers without autism. Although this hyper-awareness can lead to feelings of overwhelm, especially in people who are sensitive to loud sounds or specific types of sound, their sensitivity to sound can be used to support and simplify their processing (Remington & Fairnie, 2017). The way that Phoebe 'draws' the vocal patterns may be one way of helping maintain a focus on vocal sounds and social rhythms when there is a lot of sensory information to take in. Additionally, she reduces verbal communication to rhythm and pitch, stripped of its linguistic and segmental content. This helps simplify the auditory signal, making it easier to attend to and process.

The approach used in Intensive Interaction relies on using our earliest communicative instincts to form a relationship. Any practitioner who has learned to attend to the non-verbal cues can exploit music to start this early connection: examples are found on the Sounds of Intent (SOI) website of how practitioners use the child's sounds and early communication as a starting point for musical play and for developing attention to sound, turn-taking rhythms and vocalization. These approaches work well with children and young adults with complex needs, profound needs, limited mobility and sensory impairments. In addition to encouraging enjoyment and musical expression, the approach helps build relationships, draw attention to sound and promote an interest in others.

Once a child or young person can engage in social turn-taking through music or other interpersonal rhythms, we can begin to develop the skills of attention and precision, and engagement skills that underpin the principles of transfer from the musical domain to language (OPERA, Patel, 2011, 2014 – see Chapter 1). However, difficulties in integrating multiple sensory streams can affect social communication and verbal learning: this is something we began to explore in Chapter 2 when we examined the effect on motor timing of a mismatch between auditory and somatosensory signals in people with hearing loss and proprioceptive difficulties. These difficulties can affect social behaviour, movement and skill development. We may need to pay attention to how these skills develop and make further adjustments to how and what we teach.

Sensory integration and rhythmic flow

When we talk, dance or make music, we rely on perceiving and regulating our movement and monitoring our position in space. Our brain makes sense of incoming signals from our sensory and motor systems and integrates them: if the signals are altered or mistimed, we can exhibit unusual rhythmic behaviour. Some people with *autism*, *ADHD*, *dyspraxia* or *dyslexia* experience altered sensory processing and sensory integration. Their sensory experience affects their movement and timing and their ability to understand and use social rhythms. For example, some people with *autism, ADHD* or *dyslexia* cannot control their movements in the way they intend. Such difficulties have been called *temporo-spatial processing disorder (TSPD) of multisensory flows*. The example below from Robledo, Donnellan and Strandt-Conroy (2012) depicts the experience of an adult with autism as she learned to dance.

> I tried to learn a very simple line dance. I could not learn my footsteps and my hand movements at the same time. I had to teach my feet how to do it then stand still. I had to hold on to a rail, teach my feet their steps then lean against the wall with my feet out balancing me and learn my arm steps. Then hold on to the bar and learn my torso steps and then from there you learn what to do with the hips. Slowly, I turn the music on slow and I very, very, very slowly start the feet and very slowly add the hands then very, very slowly add the torso, etc. Everything has to be thought out, that is what is so

annoying. There are just a very few things that I do two things at the same time without thinking them through as I am going. (Geneva, aged 57, in Robledo *et al.*, 2012, p.6)

TSPD arises when multiple systems within the brain and body fail to communicate effectively, especially in the timing of signals. Geneva's account illustrates why movement with TPSD can be draining on attention and cognitive processes, at least until motor memory is established. If our body's own system fails to work in synchrony, we find it much harder to synchronize with other people or events in our environment. We will find it more difficult, still, when we are performing more than one cognitive or motor task at a time. As Geneva notes, dual tasks, such as coordinating feet *and* hands, are incredibly challenging. This requires integrating sensory information from multiple body parts and the environment. Dual motor tasks such as walking and talking can reduce our cognitive resources and performance. These types of difficulty are linked to sensory processing differences, which are also commonly found in people with *ADHD*, *dyslexia* and *dyspraxia*. The additional processing that dual tasks place on us, combined with processing differences and delays, can reduce motor coordination and accuracy in timing and movement, increase processing time and cause apparent clumsiness.

The consequences of poor sensory integration apply to social interactions, as well as to movements. When communicating with another, we must process multiple senses, and interference to one or more sensory signals can affect how we learn verbal and non-verbal communication. For example, an infant attempting to mimic a speech sound such as /b/ (as in 'book') must process and integrate:

- visual signals relating to the positioning of the lips, jaw and muscles
- the movement of these as the sound is released
- the changes in sound that characterize a /b/ from its initial 'stopped' silence through to a relatively loud 'plosive' pop that occurs as the vocal folds briefly oscillate and the breath releases, before the sound diminishes into breath and silence.

When listening to someone talk, we must also make sense of the rapidly shifting sensory data from syllables, words, gestures, intonation, voice quality and facial expressions. If we wish to respond, we must coordinate our internally generated voice and speech systems and vocalize at just the right time. If we speak too early, we interrupt the other person; too late, and we risk interrupting or losing our turn. Faced with this complexity of interactions, it is clear why sensory integration is essential for communication, interaction and movement.

Difficulties in sensory integration can make movement difficult, especially with people and objects, but movement is essential to help children and young people begin to make sense of their world. Movement-based activities can be designed that challenge and stimulate multiple senses. With appropriate stimulation and practice, the nervous system learns how to process and make meaning of the signals from its senses, and, over time, the young person learns to change their physiological or behavioural response. Music-based movement has been used successfully by occupational therapists and music therapists to support sensory integration in people with *ADHD* and with *autism* (e.g. Berger, 2002). As explored in Chapter 2, multiple sensory signals must be integrated when we step or tap to the pulse. For example, when stepping and clapping to the beat, we might integrate vestibular, proprioceptive, auditory and visual senses. Although we cannot directly observe sensory needs, a music therapist or occupational therapist can identify possible problems. A music therapist with knowledge of sensory integration can help create tasks that address specific areas of difficulty, including audio-visual integration, auditory-physical integration, and planning for movements based on auditory-visual information. To the young person with sensory challenges, the world can appear disjointed and frightening, but:

> For the brain, information paced by rhythmic pulse and pattern is non-threatening. As soon as information becomes structured and organized within rhythm and pitch patterns, which the brain prefers to process rather than random items, fear disappears and the brain allows the opening of passages to higher channels of cognition. (Berger, 2002, p.117)

Please see Berger (in 'Recommended reading') to learn more about the role of music therapy for children with autism and sensory integration difficulties.

How do ADHD and autism affect speech rhythm?

Unsurprisingly, children and young people with sensory integration difficulties, including ADHD or autism, often exhibit differences in verbal turn-taking and social synchrony. For example, children with ADHD can have timing difficulties in oral communication: they might mistime their response, leading to sudden interruptions or a failure to respond (Tannock, 2018; Nielson, 2017). Children and young adults with autism and ADHD can also have impaired perception of speech rhythm. Slow or altered sound processing is associated with autism and ADHD (Riccio *et al.*, 1994). This can make it difficult for them to accurately perceive the energy changes that help us track syllables and speech sounds. People with autism and ADHD may also have differences in *executive function*, which affect listening skills and self-regulation (e.g. Barkley, 2011, 2022). Consequently, some young people might find it hard to track rhythms in speech due to difficulties attending to the signal or filtering out environmental or competing noise.

Most children with ADHD do not have difficulty producing rhythmic speech at the syllabic level, despite the enhanced risk of perceptual or attentional difficulties. However, some children with ADHD display altered speech (Tannock, 2018). For example, they might speak with subtle phonological differences, they might develop some speech sounds later than their neurotypical peers, and they have an increased risk of stuttering, as formulating speech needs both attention and working memory, which can be compromised by ADHD. Difficulties in sensory processing and integration can also negatively affect speech articulation: clear, fluent speech relies on us receiving, integrating and making sense of signals from our articulators, as well as from our ears. These effects on speech perception and production may not affect all children or young people with ADHD, but they help explain an increased risk of dyslexia in people with ADHD (Boada, Willcutt & Pennington, 2012). It is not an easy task to learn the symbols for speech sounds if the speech sounds are poorly perceived.

It seems that people with autism can find it harder to process speech sounds than musical sounds. Haesen, Boets and Wagemans (2011) summarize data from many neurological studies investigating the perception of speech and non-speech sound in people with autism. They concluded that a sub-group use their brain's right hemisphere to process timbral and temporal aspects of sound, whereas most adults use their brain's left hemisphere. Haesen *et al.* (2011) argue that a less efficient or less involved left hemisphere explains why some people with autism have problems processing rapid temporal aspects of speech. These results were reported only in people with autism who also have language delay and may not apply to people with more advanced language skills. Similar results are reported in people with *developmental language disorder*. Finally, there is evidence that people with autism process single features and detail of sounds well but might not be able to put these details together to form a cohesive picture. For example, they might process the pitch, loudness, timbre or rhythm in a stressed word, but they do not integrate these dimensions into a *single* sound unit.

Any difficulties in perceiving speech rhythm will impact rhythmic production. Many people with autism speak with subtly different prosody compared to neurotypical peers. A recent study with adults diagnosed with autism identified differences in the stress patterns of four-syllable words (Kargas *et al.*, 2016). The adults in the study used atypical pitch, intensity and duration to mark stressed syllables. Differences were more apparent in individuals who were least sensitive to word stress: their speech seemed too fast, too slow or unusual in intonation or stress. The results confirm that problems in detecting speech rhythm lead to noticeable differences when speaking for young people with autism.

Motor-rhythm skills in autism and ADHD

Despite an increased risk of sensory and motor difficulties affecting timing, most people with *autism* or *ADHD* have well-developed music skills. As observed in Chapter 2, some children with *ADHD* have problems in beat entrainment. However, there is no evidence of a specific motor-timing deficit: a study published in 2018 showed that rhythm skills were not affected in children and adolescents with ADHD, despite weak metrical perception (Nunez-Silva *et al.*, 2018). However, sensory integration deficits can interfere with precise motor-auditory timing for rhythms and make the learner more vulnerable to rhythmic difficulties.

A few children and adults with autism have extraordinary musical skills, such as the pianist Derek Paravicini. Although blind, with autism and severe learning disabilities, Derek plays with technical precision and creativity (Ockelford, 2013). Such abilities are uncommon, though, and according to Ockelford, they arise from the unique interaction between having both autism and being blind. Most people with autism have musical-motor skills that develop in line with their non-verbal cognitive abilities, and their age. Atypical motor functions do not affect motor skills for music. A child with autism who displays motor behaviours that co-occur with autism – such as poor postural control, poor bilateral coordination, walking on tiptoes – might perform rhythmic music tasks to the same ability as their neurotypical peers, or better. Similarly, rhythmic music skills do not change as the number or severity of autism symptoms increases (Jamey *et al.*, 2019). However, children who have autism and developmental delays perform less well in rhythmic tasks such as clapping, and their ability to synchronize with another person is often poor. Also, some have difficulties discriminating metrical accent in tests that use a simple acoustic signal, such as a pure tone, or single pitched instrument. It may be less easy to discriminate rhythm from a complex acoustic signal, such as speech, or to discriminate rhythm from a piece of music that has multiple rhythms and timbres.

Summary: Using music for rhythm in people with social, sensory and attentional differences

Sensory-based difficulties can affect social communication and speech. The 'large' social rhythms are necessary precursors to developing verbal skills; however, children and adults with sensory integration difficulties can struggle to make sense of these, especially when their own movement and timing are affected. Additionally, children with autism and ADHD can have trouble attending to speech. Auditory processing difficulties can affect how well sounds and syllables are perceived and stored, attentional differences can affect processing for speech, and complex sound signals may be harder to process. Rhythm can support interpersonal communication, sensory integration and perception of temporal rhythms at different scales despite these difficulties. Making music with others can develop interpersonal rhythm skills, such as early communication skills like turn-taking, shared attention or simply being with another and sharing rhythmic movement. Games and songs can prompt a turn for vocalizing or filling a gap with an action or sound. Music is a powerful tool for supporting multisensory integration, especially when combined with movement. As music therapist and sensory integration specialist Dorita S. Berger writes: 'Any rhythmic music task that incorporates physical participation can aid rhythm internalisation. A predominance of drumming and rhythmic movement is highly recommended' (Berger, 2002, pp.155–156).

Many studies show how musical rhythm activities can support skills that underpin communication and speech in children and young people with autism. Music can also support communication in people with ADHD; but as most children with ADHD have clear speech production, we might want to use music to help them attend to speech, and the different layers of rhythm. As we saw in Chapter 2, a steady rhythmic beat can support multiple attentional skills, including sustained attention, selective attention and the ability to switch attention. Even non-isochronous rhythms in music and language have a guiding rhythmic structure that helps the brain predict when certain events will occur – this is the principle of 'neural oscillation' in the PRISM hypothesis (Chapter 3). A rhythmic structure can help children with autism and ADHD to maintain attention to speech-based rhythms. Some researchers argue that improvements in speech following musical-rhythmic intervention may be a sign of improved sensory integration (Bharathi *et al.*, 2019). In Chapter 5, we will review practical activities to support these skills.

SECTION 2: DIFFERENCES AND DIFFICULTIES IN MOTOR-BASED RHYTHMS

Above, we have looked at some examples of how rhythmic timing is affected by difficulties in making sense of the rhythms we perceive and feel – in such 'bottom-up' processing, the brain has problems understanding incoming information or signals from our body. This section looks at examples of motor difficulties that arise from disrupted brain-to-body – or 'top-down' – communication: stuttering, cluttering and dyspraxia/apraxia of speech.

Stuttering and *cluttering* are fluency disorders. Stuttering tends to affect syllables, sounds and monosyllabic words. The speaker might hesitate or repeat a sound or word, or the sounds become stuck or 'blocked', so the speaker cannot produce them. In cluttering, the rhythm of speech is affected: speech might appear overly fast, words or syllables may seem to run into each other, and syllables may be omitted. Stuttering and cluttering can occur in people with *ADHD*, *autism* and *developmental delays*. The cause of these fluency disorders is uncertain. Many suggest that stuttering arises from a central deficit in motor timing (e.g. Falk, Müller & Dalla-Bella, 2014), which might stem from delayed or altered sensory feedback. Others argue that people who stutter have a poorer perception of rhythm, but this, too, is debated. Although a timing deficit might contribute to stuttering, psychological and cognitive factors are important, too, for both stuttering and cluttering. For example, cluttering can occur when the speech system cannot keep up with thoughts, and stuttering is heightened by anxiety.

Whereas a fluency disorder affects the rhythmic flow of speech, *verbal apraxia/dyspraxia* affects how clearly someone forms speech sounds. People with verbal apraxia/dyspraxia have problems making movements for speech. The muscles are undamaged, but the brain sometimes gives them the wrong instructions. The child knows what they want to say, but the messages to the muscles go awry, leading to poorly timed muscular movements or sequences of movement. Specialists attribute the cause of dyspraxia to areas in the brain that are specialized for motor planning and timing. Dyspraxia can affect non-verbal movements and speech, which hints at a widespread difficulty in sequencing and programming rhythmic movements.

The primary cause of dyspraxia is not weak muscles, but a child or adult can have dyspraxia with *dysarthria*, which is caused by damaged or weakened muscles that affect voice and speech. The symptoms of *dyspraxia* and *dysarthria* can be similar. Both conditions affect speech timing at different temporal levels. At small temporal levels, a child with these conditions will find it hard to form speech sounds clearly, and they may mispronounce words. They will have problems with timing for rhythmic phrases and syllables at larger temporal levels. For example, they might lengthen or shorten syllables, pause their speech, omit syllables, or emphasize syllables or sounds incorrectly.

Dyspraxia and dysarthria commonly occur in people with *cerebral palsy* and people with *Down syndrome*. People with dyspraxia and dysarthria may experience *stuttering* and *cluttering*, too. In such complex cases – for example, those with Down syndrome – it can be challenging for clinicians to determine the cause of speech difficulties, especially when multiple additional factors are involved, such as *hearing impairment*, *sensory processing or integration difficulties*, *cognitive difficulties*, and difficulties in *speech perception*. However, as we will see later in this chapter, music-based rhythmic activities can support motor planning and programming difficulties, such as dyspraxia and stuttering. Rhythmic music also holds promise for helping speech in learners who have multiple needs.

We will now examine rhythm in people with Down syndrome. Below, I discuss some of the challenges they can face with motor timing in speech and music and how music can support their ability to perceive and make speech-based rhythms. Many children and young people can have motor-based difficulties in making accurate rhythmic movements for speech or music, which can arise from muscular weaknesses, motor-programming or planning deficits, or from neurological disorders. However, the difficulties that can hamper speech and music in people with Down syndrome are similar to those in other groups, despite different causes.

Rhythmic skills in people with Down syndrome

People with Down syndrome have long been described as musical and having good rhythmic skills. However, multiple factors can affect their speech: dyspraxia, muscle weakness, auditory processing disorder, altered proprioception, stuttering and cluttering, and, for a sub-group, ADHD and autism. Despite this constellation of complicating issues, people with Down syndrome can develop good motor-timing skills in music, offering considerable potential for supporting speech perception and production in people with Down syndrome and people with less complex needs.

RHYTHMIC SPEECH PERCEPTION IN PEOPLE WITH DOWN SYNDROME

People with Down syndrome are likely to have difficulties perceiving word rhythm, even when hearing loss and poor auditory-verbal memory abilities are accounted for. As young children, their perception of some rhythmic structures is delayed compared to those without Down syndrome (Mason-Apps, Stojanovic & Houston-Price, 2011). In Standard English, most nouns emphasize the first syllable (see also Chapter 3). For example, the word 'city' has a strong first syllable; but the word 'settee' has a weak initial syllable. Weak initial words are less common in Standard English. Children with Down syndrome have problems perceiving such weakly stressed syllables at the beginning of words. A study revealed that children and adolescents with Down syndrome (aged 11–20 years) had difficulties discriminating and repeating nonsense words with simple and complex stress patterns (Pettinato & Verhoeven, 2009). The participants with Down syndrome also had difficulty reproducing syllables as the target syllable length increased. Their speech became less accurate in longer words and 'weak' syllable positions, such as words with *weak-strong* stress patterns. The authors concluded that children with Down syndrome do not easily encode these types of speech rhythm and that they acquire these complex speech rhythms later than most children. This can cause them problems in perceiving complex word rhythms in continuous speech. This will affect their abilities to perceive some words and reproduce words that have more complex rhythmic structures.

RHYTHMIC SPEECH PRODUCTION IN PEOPLE WITH DOWN SYNDROME

Most children and adults with Down syndrome have problems acquiring and using rhythmic speech. Their perceptual, physical and cognitive factors can all affect speech development. For example, fluctuating levels of *hearing loss* can interfere with the acquisition of speech sounds; reduced *auditory memory* may limit storage and retrieval of sounds; *hypermobility* and *poor proprioception* reduce strength and accuracy of oro-motor movements; and difficulties in *phonation* (see Chapter 7) and control of *respiration* (see Chapter 6) can affect the distinction between paired voiced/unvoiced speech sounds (e.g. b/p, d/t) and reduce control of pitch, duration or intensity. Someone with Down syndrome might also have difficulties articulating speech sounds because of anatomical and dental features, including teeth gaps, occlusion or a high palatal vault. Many learners with Down syndrome can reproduce speech sounds and oro-motor movements in isolation, but they can have difficulty implementing these in their speech.

The examples below show some characteristics of speech rhythm in two young people with Down syndrome who took part in my research. Each had a very different voice and speech style – although each could sing fluently and articulate speech sounds clearly in single words, their speech would change when they became excited, when they became anxious or when there were high demands on their cognitive processes. For example, when asked to repeat a sentence or a novel word, they would show increasing dysfluency, and their voices would become more dysphonic (see Chapter 7). The first example below (Figure 4.1) shows an extract from a conversation with Rachel. She emphasized some syllables strongly (Gert, good, brill, times, fact) but her speaking rate was uneven; some syllables seemed to collide, some sounds were missing, and her sounds were unclear. Her intonational contour and emphasis on specific syllables communicated her meaning more clearly than the speech sounds, and it was my knowledge of the context in which she spoke that helped me interpret her meaning.

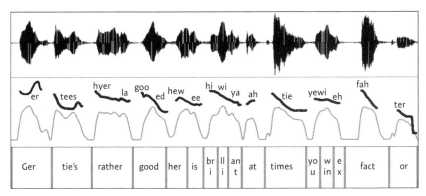

Figure 4.1: Rachel's spontaneous speech. The top image layer of the shows the waveform; the next layer shows the pitch (dark grey line) with a representation of her speech articulation and the changes in intensity (lighter grey line). Rachel emphasized the syllables marked in bold, as she said '**Ger**tie's rather **good**. She is **brill**iant at **times**. You win ex-**fac**tor'. Like many young people with Down syndrome, some speech sounds were unclear or missing but she used rhythmic stress and pitch well to help her communicate.

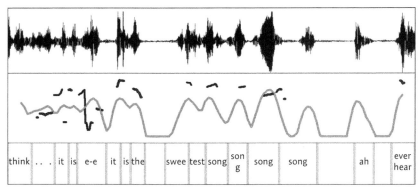

Figure 4.2: Spontaneous speech from Andrew. There were multiple hesitations and repetitions in this short phrase as Andrew tried to finish what he wanted to say. This affected the rhythm of his speech. Additionally, his voice was dysphonic, which meant he could not easily control his pitch or the intensity of his speech.

The second example, above, shows a comment made by Andrew. His voice was usually dysphonic, making it hard for him to use his voice – for this reason, the pitch contour (dark line, Figure 4.2) is broken, rather than smooth, like Rachel's. When he used short sentences or sang, his articulation was clear and his speech was fluent and appropriately rhythmic. However, he struggled when he wanted to produce a complex sentence. His words appeared 'blocked', and he repeated whole words (*the*, *song*). At times, he would audibly grind his teeth or make sounds of frustration when he could not produce his intended words. Go to Video 3 in the online resources to see and hear these two samples.

Musical-rhythmic skills in people with Down syndrome

People with Down syndrome are often described as having good rhythmic skills and being keen and able dancers. Unless they have a *dual diagnosis* of autism or severe learning disabilities, they do not have the same types of social synchrony difficulties as you notice in some people with autism or with ADHD. However, their physiological differences, such as low muscle tone, *hypermobility* and reduced *proprioception*, can affect the timing, consistency and speed of their motor movements. Over the past 50 years, several studies have provided detail about their motor-rhythmic skills in musical tasks, which confirm some differences compared to other groups. Early research identified that children and young adolescents with Down syndrome had some difficulties making rhythmic movements to music (Stratford & Ching, 1989). Compared to children with similar cognitive abilities, those with Down syndrome were less accurate as they 'hammered', marched and clapped to the music. However, they scored more highly on 'butterfly' movements than children in the control group. The authors concluded that the group with Down syndrome had a sense of musical timing but that motoric limitations hampered them in some movements.

More detailed information about the rhythmic skills of children and adults with Down syndrome was given by a music therapist delivering community music and music therapy sessions across a range of regions from Wales and the West of England. Picard (2009) documented the rhythmic characteristics of people with Down syndrome of varying ages, from toddlers to old-age pensioners. When commenting on structured call-and-response activities, in which participants were required to clap back rhythmic patterns, Picard wrote that the rhythmic production was 'relatively accurate' but that responses were inaccurate in the onset of their timing relative to the beat. She noted that in this session, and others, some participants with Down syndrome responded sooner than required – sometimes, before the rhythm had been fully demonstrated – while others reacted later. Individuals were also inconsistent in the timing of responses relative to the beat. Despite the poor alignment of rhythms, Picard deemed that the rhythmic reproduction of most people she observed was accurate.

Picard did not use audio or video to record the call-and-response patterns, so we cannot be sure how out of time the responses were or what range of possible factors may have led to this. However, I noticed similar patterns in some of my students and research participants. I examined rhythmic accuracy in four adults across various tasks (Jeffery, 2016). I studied how closely their movements aligned with the rhythm and how well they reproduced the intervals between movements as they danced, walked and clapped to music; entrained to a rhythm; clapped the rhythm of a song. Participants were asked to do this on their own (auditory only) to begin with; but were given visual support to help them if they seemed to need it (demonstration, accompaniment, graphic notation). The four adults were similar in age and cognitive ability but differed in their speech and rhythmic skills. Kerry and Robert were extreme opposites. Kerry could accurately repeat some rhythmic patterns and independently clapped the words of a song. When imitating clapped patterns, the duration between Kerry's claps was accurate if the number of *beats* did not exceed her digit span (three to four); for example, she could repeat seven claps that were 'chunked' over a bar of four beats (e.g. *tee-tee, tee-tee, ta, tee-tee*). However, she could not repeat the whole pattern if the rhythmic patterns exceeded four beats or included triplets (e.g. *ti-ri-ti, ta, tee-tee, ta*).

Kerry's musical skills were more highly developed than her verbal skills suggested. She could entrain to a rhythm, a skill that grows at about ten years of age, but her skills in using words were roughly equivalent to a child of about three to four years. In contrast, Robert could not perceive rhythmic patterns independently; even when given visual support, he struggled to make clear, consistent rhythmic movements.

The reasons for differences in rhythmic motor movements in people with Down syndrome are complex. As explored in Chapter 2, they depend in part on the interactions between *hearing acuity*, *auditory memory capacity*, *auditory processing abilities* and the amount of *practice*; and on issues such as *dyspraxia*, *weak muscle tone* and *proprioception*. Although motor difficulties are commonly delayed in people with Down syndrome, there is considerable evidence that they can improve strength, coordination and agility. Therefore, we can be confident that we can help them improve the *precision* of their timing in music (which works towards the 'P' of the OPERA (Patel, 2011, 2014) hypothesis). To help them learn, we must consider how we reduce the impacts of their hearing loss, processing and physical differences. Their musical rhythmic skills will improve if they are not straining to hear, perceive or remember the pattern. Visual teaching methods are especially successful in improving accuracy.

Using music to support motor-speech difficulties

Music therapists have been using rhythmic activities to support speech motor difficulties for a long time. While therapists work with children who have complex speech needs, the research typically involves people who have just one type of speech disorder or one that is recently acquired; for example, people with *dysarthria*, or people who have lost their speech following a stroke, brain injury or Parkinson's disease. Their research has shown that rhythmic training in speech can make significant differences for some people (e.g. Thaut, 2005). Specialized programmes such as Rhythmic Speech Cueing (RSC) are proven to support speech recovery and promote speech intelligibility in people with acquired speech problems. RSC uses a treatment plan that develops according to the individual's needs. It might begin with metrical cues, in which someone learns to speak syllables or words in time to a beat at a tempo that best suits them; they might then learn to speak text or poems to a beat. Rhythmic patterns that emulate natural speech might be used: the patient might learn to say phrases in time with a rhythm that includes stress markers. These types of activities can gradually improve or restore natural-sounding speech. This approach draws on extensive neurological and motor research (e.g. Thaut, 2005) but requires clinical oversight.

This type of rhythmic therapy has promise for verbal dyspraxia and speech dysfluencies (Mainka & Mallien, 2014). Even simple activities – such as speaking to an audible beat – can have a significant impact. Neurological studies suggest that people who stutter have increased difficulty integrating sensorimotor information and planning rhythmic movements. The presence of an audible beat or rhythm in music might make up for this difficulty – it provides a motor plan that 'compensates' for the differences in brain function and helps focus attention (Frankford *et al.*, 2021).

Given the complexity of speech perception and production, you might wonder whether musical activities will make any difference to young people with lifelong difficulties. The answer is a qualified 'yes'. The speech system is vulnerable in conversational speech, which requires linguistic planning. Cognitive load or stress interferes with speech production so that a child might make excellent progress in single words or phrases, but – like Andrew – they might struggle when using them in conversation. Nevertheless, we can do much to support the perception of speech rhythms and the rhythmic production of words and phrases. Rhythmic priming can help children and young people perceive syllables for words; slower production of speech sounds in rhythms and poems can assist perception of speech sounds; and learning words and phrases in a rhythmic context can help focus attention. Rhythmic priming may be significant for helping children with Down syndrome to hear and process weakly stressed syllables – the rhythmic structure of such words can be emphasized through rhythm activities (e.g. making the syllable louder) and singing.

Rhythmic activities may support people with Down syndrome to produce clearly articulated syllables in words; with enough practice, they can strengthen the rhythmic templates for words and speech sounds. This approach may benefit those with dysfluencies, such as stuttering or cluttering. Practising words and phrases to a steady rhythm can help support intelligibility, reduce speaking rate, and reduce anxiety around speaking words, which can exacerbate dysfluency. If children and young people practise producing error-free words and phrases in a music-based context, they might be able to reproduce them more easily in speech. This is an idea we will return to in Chapter 9, when we examine singing for speech, and in Chapter 10, when we look at the transfer of learning to speech.

CHAPTER SUMMARY

The factors that support the perception and production of rhythm in music and speech are complex. A child or young adult might have sensory differences that alter how they perceive movements and sounds. They might have rhythmic motor differences that affect limbs, speech and voice, or muscle weaknesses that impair movements.

Some children and young people, such as those with autism, can have difficulties making sense of rhythm in movement and social situations. They might have a poor sense of their own motor or verbal rhythms, and they may process or perceive sounds and movement in ways that we cannot directly know. However, we can be alert to their rhythmic movements and responses and use these as a bridge to connect; we can simplify the verbal signal, or augment it to support perception, attention and processing. Music can support the development of social rhythms by emphasizing turn-taking and providing clear structure, routine and a sense of control. Additionally, music can support sensory integration and make it easier for some learners to process multiple streams of stimuli.

Given that many people with autism and ADHD have reasonable limb-motor control for music, their motor skills can be exploited to develop an awareness of speech rhythms, which can be an area of difficulty. Difficulties in speech rhythm may be more noticeable in people with motor differences, such as people with Down syndrome. People with Down syndrome have multiple barriers to overcome. Despite this, their strengths in visual processing can help them develop their motor timing difficulties and support their poor auditory-verbal processing skills.

Many children and young people can have difficulties from overlapping sensory and motor-based differences. However, once we understand some of the challenges a learner might be facing, we can develop different approaches to support rhythm skills at large and small levels. Ideas for developing rhythm skills in music and speech are given in Chapter 5.

RECOMMENDED READING

Berger, D.S. (2002), *Music Therapy, Sensory Integration and the Autistic Child*. London: Jessica Kingsley Publishers.

Cummins, F. (2015). Rhythm and Speech. In M.A. Redford (ed.), *The Handbook of Speech Production*, pp.158–177. Chichester: John Wiley & Sons.

Williams, D. (1996). *Autism – An Inside-Out Approach: An Innovative Look at the Mechanics of 'Autism' and Its Developmental Cousins*. London: Jessica Kingsley Publishers.

CHAPTER 5

Making Rhythm Work for Social Communication and Speech

THE BIG QUESTIONS

How do we support rhythm skills and adapt them to meet cognitive, learning and sensory needs? Which speech and communication skills will rhythmic music activities benefit?

By the end of this chapter, you will:

- understand how to adapt musical activities to develop different sensory and cognitive skills
- consider what other adaptations might support accuracy in motor movements for rhythm
- know how you can use songs, games and rhythmic musical activities to support rhythmic skills for speech, including:
  - turn-taking
  - perception of rhythmic structure in words
  - perception of meter and accent in music and speech
  - rhythmic and metrical production of speech.

WHO IS THIS FOR?

This chapter contains ideas that can be used with any developing child or young adult, and those with physical, sensory and cognitive differences. It provides example activities to demonstrate how to adapt activities for *postural stability*, *proprioception*, *auditory perception* and *auditory memory*. It suggests adapting activities to focus on different skills (*movement*, *attention*, *speech perception*). The later sections explore how to tailor songs, rhythm games and activities to support awareness of *speech rhythm, syllable duration, accent* and *stress*; and how to prime learning for *words* and *phrases*.

The previous chapters aimed to help you understand the similarities and differences between rhythms in language and music and show you how these skills develop for most children and learners who follow different learning pathways. We explored some of these complex issues and considered how and why music-based rhythm activities support speech perception and production. This chapter has a practical focus, but I connect practical activities with the research evidence and theory to explain how they can help. I provide some examples in this chapter to help you plan how and why you might use 'everyday' rhythm activities to support developing verbal skills. I explain how you might adapt rhythmic music activities to reduce barriers to learning – for example, to reduce the demands on working memory or to encourage greater physical control when playing. Appropriate adaptations can reduce unhelpful effort and help learners develop precision of timing. I also provide examples of how you might use activities to support various goals through a single activity, including awareness of speech rhythms, awareness of meter in music and language, social skills, using words, and musical ability and literacy.

We will begin by revisiting some general principles before exploring how to support rhythmic movement and use rhythm activities for speech.

GENERAL PRINCIPLES OF SUPPORTING RHYTHM DEVELOPMENT

We can support all children and young people to develop their early rhythm skills by consciously emulating how most children naturally develop rhythm skills in speech and music (see Chapter 3). There are five general principles we should apply:

1. Create a music-rich environment.
2. Support social rhythms.
3. Use songs, rhymes and infant-directed speech to support rhythm skills.
4. Adapt activities for age and developmental maturity.
5. Find ways to embody rhythm.

The rationale for each is explained below.

Create a music-rich environment

We need to provide a culturally diverse music environment, especially for very young children. As with speech sounds, the infant learns what sounds are relevant to their culture's music through exposure. Also, as with speech, sensitivity to rhythmic nuances may be 'lost' as the infant learns they are culturally irrelevant. In music, exposure to the complex rhythms of different cultures results in 'bimusicality', which may be equated with bilingualism. For example, a child who learns English and Japanese must master two different rules for rhythm in language: English allows for variability in duration, but Japanese uses a system where syllables and words are made up of time-based units, called 'morae'. The music of each culture may well capture these linguistic rhythms (Chapter 3). A recent study (Vaquero *et al.*, 2020) showed that long-term exposure to either music training or a second language produces changes in the brain, in the auditory pathways that connect auditory, multisensory and motor pathways. Therefore, we can argue that exposure to a wide variety of rhythms may 'work' the brain's processing capabilities similarly to early exposure to a second language. For children at risk of speech perception difficulties, being encultured in music in addition to spoken language may best support the skills needed for both speech and music.

Support social rhythms

Use songs and music games to encourage social communication's 'big' temporal rhythms. Musical and vocal activities can be used to mimic the same sort of 'peekaboo' games that are used with toddlers – the aim is to create anticipation and expectation of a response and leave a gap for the child or young person to respond. You can adapt the type of response you want to suit their development, age or ability; for example, you could accept a smile or a look as an 'answer', or a rustle of fabric, the shake of a bell, or a vocalization. As a learner becomes more verbal, you might expect them to fill in the words or finish a phrase. This type of activity has broad appeal. For example, it has helped parents/carers of children with autism to develop social communication (e.g. Way to Play, Autism NZ, New Zealand: see the box below for more about this approach). The book, *Let's All Listen* (Lloyd, 2007), has examples of rhythmic games and call-and-response songs, with suggested learning outcomes related to social communication, musical skills and language development.

Use songs, rhymes and infant-directed speech to support rhythm skills

Simple songs and infant-directed speaking styles can support perception of speech rhythm. Infant-directed speech, rhymes and simple songs exaggerate the rhythmic structure of words and phrases, and this helps infants pick out sounds, syllables, words and phrase structures. The style of infant-directed speech has been shown to support language processing, and it may be that using a similarly rhythmic form of language will continue to support processing in older children or adults who are at an earlier level of language. To suit their age and interest, you can rewrite simple-sounding songs and rhymes for older learners.

Adapt activities for age and developmental maturity

As we saw in Chapter 2, the ability to synchronize motor movements to a pulse develops slowly in infants and in line with motor maturity. Half of children at eight years of age do not have the motor control to produce a metrical accent in a steady beat. The ability to reproduce rhythm also develops slowly, in line with motor skills, cognitive skills such as attention and auditory memory, and experience. The mode of instruction and production affects performance while motor and attentional skills are developing. Children of about five years can more easily reproduce rhythms based on word syllables than tapped rhythms and may find this even easier if the rhythms are sung. Although most children have developed the skills needed for rhythm by about seven to eight years, their accuracy in skills does continue to grow with practice and maturity, and some skills – such as the ability to entrain to complex rhythms – may take a few more years to emerge. This means that children with motor-movement disorders or cognitive delays might fall behind their peers in music-making skills. However, some children and adults with learning differences have 'spiky' profiles. Like James (Chapter 1) or Georgina (Chapter 2), musical abilities may be advanced relative to other skills or areas of development.

Find ways to embody rhythm

The embodiment of rhythm means using movement to feel rhythmic patterns. This has many advantages, including developing a physical awareness of timing and patterns; integrating different senses – cognitive, sensorimotor, auditory; and giving you, an observer, an understanding of how well someone can produce and imitate movements.

Learning to move – or to be moved – in time to an aural rhythm can sharpen perception of the rhythm. Movement-based rhythm activities are commonly used to develop musicality. For example, in Dalcroze Eurhythmics, pupils walk, step, dance and pass objects in rhythmic patterns – a small step on a short note, and two long steps for more extended notes. Body percussion activities can also help create a visual and tangible experience. However, some actions will be more difficult than others to perform in time to a beat, depending on the motor skills involved and the individual's ability to see or feel their movements; if stepping in time is too hard, try 'flying' motions, drumming motions or clapping, and so on. You might need to change the type of movement a learner uses if you aim to assess their rhythm skills. In general, larger motor movements are more difficult to time accurately than smaller limb motor movements, such as tapping. Try various movements to help you understand the learner's strengths and needs; or ask them to create their own 'best' action.

WAY TO PLAY: USING MUSICAL PLAY WITH CHILDREN WITH AUTISM AND THEIR FAMILIES

Alison Taylor, lecturer in special educational needs, disability and inclusion

Way to Play is an approach developed in New Zealand that supports families of children with autism to open up communication and interaction through play, and through musical play, especially.

Musical elements of social play have helped young children with autism make genuine connections with their adults and develop words and gestures to initiate and sustain these favoured play patterns (Beaumont *et al.*, 2021). Using pattern, memory and variation, the Way to Play strategies provide familiarity, prompts and opportunities for development while engaging the child with autism in musical and playful interactions. Starting from the child's own actions, the adult can establish a pattern through repeated imitation. Children with autism can be afraid of unpredictability and spontaneity, so the pattern provides reassurance. This pattern can be marked by using rhythmic or melodic phrases which can be used to trigger memory and positive association to encourage future interaction. These can be linked to traditional songs (such as Peekaboo, King of the Castle) or by using the voice as an instrument to create a phrase relating to the activity. Once a favourite play pattern is established, the musical or linguistic 'memory catchphrase' that signals the game can become a powerful communication tool for the child to engage with and then initiate a social connection. The catchphrase also supports the creation of memories of emotion-based experiences – something which can be more challenging for children with autism to form and recall. This simple approach can reduce social stress and increase opportunities for social engagement and fun (Stuart, 2016).

Way to Play is underpinned by theory of early development of interaction. This includes social-pragmatic approaches such as those used in Intensive Interaction (Nind & Hewett, 1994), Experience Sharing (Ngan *et al.*, 2011) and Relationship Development Intervention (Gutstein, Burgess & Montfort, 2007). These approaches are evident in how practitioners use sound to build connections. In the very earliest stages of development, music and language merge as unintentional sound. As favourable responses from caregivers are forthcoming, so intentional sounds are made to elicit further favourable responses. Children begin to learn the basics of social interaction – facial expressions, vocalizations, intonation, body language and shared attention – and as these develop, increasingly conscious thought is required to sustain, extend and vary these interactions. When a carer uses Way to Play with a child with autism, they vary their own responses to the child's interaction: this introduces productive uncertainty in the form of changes that are small and still within the safe realms of the familiar and engaging play pattern. The variation aspect of Way to Play encourages the child to use their developing cognition, to go on to develop thinking and problem-solving skills. This blossoming connectiveness increases the child's attention to the adult's voice, face and movements, which is an important prerequisite of social communication.

The musical element of the Way to Play strategies makes an important contribution to its effectiveness. Stamou *et al.* (2019) identify music and dance as highly engaging for young children with autism. Their findings suggest there are also improvements in physical proximity, physical contact and cooperation, all of which are conducive to improved social communication. The repetition and pattern of music appeals to the preference for familiarity that is often experienced by those on the spectrum. When body movements and big rhythms are added to the music, non-verbal communication occurs between the people moving together. Music emphasizes social connections, encouraging shared and joint attention and providing clearly defined opportunities for engaging in turn-taking.

Music serves social, emotional and cognitive functions in everyday life and will continue to support children into adolescence and adulthood (Kirby & Burland, 2022). In their study, Kirby and Burland identified the importance of music in the lives of young people with autism. Socially, music creates connection, it offers a theme for conversation based on common music appreciation, and gives opportunities for sharing an experience of listening to music or making and performing music together. Emotionally, the connection is felt, although not always articulated. Emotional functions of music include mood management, emotional regulation, decoding emotion, emotional expression and nostalgia. Even when music is not the primary activity, its cognitive function and positive effects include motivation, enhancement of an activity, positive distraction and support for routine. If engagement through music and positive association with social connection can be achieved early on, then music can continue to support the social communication of young people with autism into adulthood.

SUPPORTING CONTROLLED MOTOR MOVEMENTS WHEN MAKING MUSIC

Before skills in rhythm can transfer to speech, a learner must accurately perceive rhythmic cues. We can use beat and rhythm to enable fluent speech and practise words and phrases. To encourage deep learning – the type that can strengthen pathways between the body and brain – we need to develop accuracy and precision when making music (see OPERA, Patel, 2011, 2014; and PRISM, Fiveash *et al.*, 2021). Where possible, we need learners to reproduce rhythms with the correct durational patterns, and align rhythmic patterns to a beat.

In sum, we want to use rhythmic motor activities to:

- develop social and communicative interaction
- support attention to and perception of durational patterns and stress cues in speech
- enable fluent, rhythmic speech production in words and phrases
- develop skills that will transfer from the musical domain to speech.

And we can best facilitate these outcomes by helping children and young people to:

- use songs and games to emphasize rhythmic structures such as turn-taking and smaller cues such as stress
- make controlled motor movements that imitate timing patterns of music and words in songs
- play, clap and/or chant, speech-based rhythms with a sense of beat.

As previously discussed (Chapter 2), movements improve physical awareness of rhythm and can be used to emphasize metrical stress and contrasts in duration (e.g. long versus short). We will return to these benefits for speech in a later section; but first, we should explore how rhythm itself can prepare learners for developing musical motor skills. Working with rhythm is a valuable means of supporting movement and gait. Patients who have impaired movement following brain damage can often recover functional skills with music. Research in rhythmic rehabilitation has shown that rhythmic prompts help the brain integrate sound and motion and help it to plan motor movements. Gradually, the brain becomes better at planning and coordinating movements (e.g. see Thaut, 2005).

Although the causes of motor timing in people with developmental needs are different from those with acquired brain injury, we can apply the same principles. LaGasse and Hardy (2013) explain why some forms of rhythm-based music therapy can help people with *autism* develop greater precision in movement. They argue that external rhythmic cues (such as pulse or rhythm) facilitate motor planning and motor timing: the auditory cue assists with planning when to move. It also reduces the need to rely on proprioceptive feedback, which can be poor in many individuals with autism and other needs. Rhythmic cues can support motor functions such as gait, or other movements if the rhythm is timed to the individual's needs, but the authors also stress that other cues, such as pitch and accent, may be needed. Rhythmic singing can also be used to support some motor skills, and this includes the additional cues of pitch and stress. Research with children with *cerebral palsy* (Levin *et al.*, 2017) showed that if they sang a song of their choice to themselves as they arose from a chair and walked, their movements were faster and more coordinated than if they hadn't been singing.

We can help children and young people move with greater ease and rhythmic timing by providing a rhythmic structure at a pace that suits them. Ideally, we would encourage learners to use gross and fine motor skills when they move to a rhythm. However, we might need to be selective. Some children and young people will find it difficult to concentrate on producing movements that are accurate in timing while also maintaining postural stability. Therefore, we may need to consider additional adaptations. For example, as we have discussed, sensory integration difficulties can affect rhythmic movement and coordination in people with ADHD or autism. Hypermobility is present in all people with *Down syndrome*, and it has a high probability of affecting people with *autism* and *ADHD*: this can cause proprioceptive difficulties and muscle weaknesses. For some people with hypermobile conditions (e.g. with *Ehlers Danlos syndrome*), associated conditions such as postural orthostatic tachycardia syndrome (POTS) can cause dizziness. Some people will also have weak muscles and poorer muscular control because of neurological differences, such as *cerebral palsy*. Ideally, you will work with a physiotherapist or similar to support movement for musical activities, especially if there are confirmed physical or sensory needs. However, there are some approaches you could use to encourage accuracy and precision in movement in music-based motor tasks:

- **Encourage the young person to become aware of their posture or movement** for part of a session. For example, support them in sitting or standing with physical or tactile prompts. Aim to help them maintain this for short periods of focused learning, then allow relaxation breaks (see Video 10 in the online resources for an example). It can be challenging for some people to focus simultaneously on the movement they are making (e.g. clapping a phrase) and their posture or use of their limbs as they make these movements. Verbal cues can help them self-correct periodically once they have been taught the target posture or movement.

- **Increase or support somatosensory feedback.** Some people receive low signals from their body to their brain. Depending on the needs and wishes of the individual, you could use touch to support movement; you could use compression clothing to increase the strength of the signal from their body; you could use Kinesio tape to support a joint to stay in its ideal position and increase somatosensory feedback. These can help maintain and support posture for movement and reduce processing demands. This can give the learner more 'space' to focus on the task.
- **Use different limb-motor movements and adjust pace.** Although walking to rhythms can help internalize them, this may pose challenges to balance and stability. If using the whole body for rhythmic movements, experiment with pace and music to find one that works best for the individual – too slow a tempo can support the learner to become more aware of their motion, but could increase instability; too fast a tempo may improve stability but increase error. It may be helpful to use smaller limbs – arms/hands – for internalizing faster movement, and large motor movements, such as walking, for slower rhythms.
- **Find a type of movement that works best.** This depends on the motor skills involved and the individual's ability to see or feel their actions. If stepping in time is too hard, try 'flying' motions, drumming motions or clapping, and so on. An advantage of this type of learning is that the people you work with can create their own movements and routines.
- **Consider using graphic scores to enhance the perception of the intended rhythm.** For example, a sequence of long and short lines can show big/small steps; animal images may represent 'slow' or 'big' steps, versus shorter 'trotting' movements. Visual images can support the perception of duration in those who need more processing time or have weak auditory perception. These can be helpful precursors to learning rhythm syllables and notation. (See Video 5 in the online resources for an example of simple rhythm notation.)

USING RHYTHM MOTOR SKILLS FOR SPEECH

This section will provide examples for using rhythmic activities to support the perception of speech sounds, syllables and words in speech and to prepare learners for playing, speaking or singing rhythmic words and phrases. We need to develop perception before production, so most activities focus on how to use rhythm activities to advance a learner's perception of, for example, syllabic structures or stress. Most of the activities I suggest will allow you to include non-verbal learners as well as verbal children and adults.

Some activities require dual-motor activities (walking and talking) or the ability to divide attention (e.g. layering sounds so that one plays against another). We might want to increase the challenge for some learners: for example, we might ask for greater precision when playing or speaking a rhyme, or we could introduce a second motor task, such as clapping the beat while chanting a rhyme. Alternatively, activities can be simplified to reduce processing demands and increase focus. For example, you might reduce the number of movements you ask a learner to use; you might revert to the beat or to one level of the beat (see Chapter 2); you could direct attention to just one aspect of activity, such as timing or synchronization; or you might offer headphones or noise blockers to help a learner filter out extraneous noise and information.

Using music to prepare for verbal production of words and phrases

Many rhythm-based musical activities can support speech perception and production: below are just a few examples. Most activities show how you might develop skills in attending to and perceiving rhythms and accents in words and phrases. However, you can ask learners to perform these activities, too: this might help you assess their awareness of meter, accent and rhythm. For example, a child might show you the metrical accent even if they cannot speak with a metrical accent; or you can deliberately play with the wrong rhythm or wrong stress and let them protest, even if they cannot themselves play or speak with the necessary motor control to show accent or stress.

DRUMMING AND PERCUSSION ACTIVITIES

Words and phrases can be used as the basis for complex pieces of music in drumming circles and samba bands. These types of rhythm activities work for one-to-one sessions or groups; they can be kept simple by having all or most members of a group playing the same rhythm, or they can be used to encourage higher-level attentional skills, for example by asking a learner or group to play against another rhythm, or to alternate between patterns on cue. Images can be used to create a visual score, which can also help improve the perception of rhythmic duration and reduce cognitive load.

Different ways of performing word-based rhythms can also be used to target broader communication skills. Examples are given below and in the online resources – see especially Video series 7, and Video 10.

Call-and-response phrases

- Caller: I've got a dog
- Response: A great big dog!

Depending on the individual's goals and abilities, you can use the activity to emphasize speech articulation and meaning or support verbal turn-taking skills. For example, you can encourage group members to write their own calls and responses, enabling them to use words meaningfully and discover the rhythms of the words and phrases they know and use. Almost any phrase pair will do if each can fit into the same tempo and meter.

Layering rhythm patterns

We can create quite complex pieces of rhythmic music by 'layering' words and phrases. Such rhythm sequences can be attractive ways to embed speech therapy targets for verbal learners. For example, you can select words, sounds or nonsense syllables that align closely with an individual's speech articulation needs. You can begin with words they know and use, then introduce new words, or words with more complex syllable structures; you could focus on teaching the meaning of words; encourage the use of names, and so on.

This type of rhythm activity can include learners with diverse rhythmic, motor, musical and linguistic abilities; for example, a young person with limited mobility could play one-word syllables and keep the pulse, or play every other pulse, or a learner with well-developed motor skills could perform the type of weak-strong or compound word rhythm that can be hard for some learners to perceive (see Chapter 7). If they demonstrate these rhythms to the group, they show their skills to you and the group, or you can present the appropriate rhythm to the group to support and enhance their perception of complex rhythms.

A food-based example is below:

- Layer 1, rhythm 1: pulse – one-word syllables 'ta', e.g. Bread x 4
- Layer 2, rhythm 2: two-word syllable, 'tee-tee', e.g. Butter x 4
- Layer 3, rhythm 3: three-word syllable, 'tee-tee ta', e.g. Marmalade x 2

There are multiple ways to use activities like this. Before you begin to play percussion, you might place the target words and associated images on a board; you can ask learners to watch you clap the word, and ask them to tell you which word it is you are playing. You can prime words for speech by clapping the rhythm and asking them to clap back; clapping with the word, and asking them to clap back; asking them to say the word; asking them to think and clap the word.

When you are ready to play, you can experiment with how to use the word rhythms. You might begin with layer 1, then bring in layer 2, then layer 3. Or each rhythm can be played in sequence and played in a cycle: 1, 2, 3; 1, 2, 3. You could then divide the group, and each sub-group plays the cycle as a canon, with sub-group two coming in as group one begin rhythm 3.

The activities could be used to encourage attention to timbre; for example, you might assign a different type of instrument to each word. Or you might practise using other senses and social skills; for example, you can allocate a student or pair of students a specific rhythm and ask a conductor to decide who plays and when. The conductor can use gestures, images, sound, eye gaze and touch to start and stop individuals or groups.

You can also teach short phrases that can signal a change of activity. Some drumming traditions use distinctive rhythmic phrases as 'breaks' and cues to start and stop. My group's favourite 'break' was a call-and-response pattern. The leader would call a phrase, and the group would respond verbally and using instruments, then by internalizing the words and performing the rhythms only. An example we used is:

- Leader: Are you ready?
- Group: Yes, we are
- All: OK...let's go!

In the early stages, the leader can call the words; later, when we have learned and internalized the pattern of the words, we can use the rhythm alone. When the group is familiar with the distinctive pattern, we can use it to encourage attention to the leader, promote social awareness, practise turn-taking, 'refresh' attention and use executive function skills such as switching focus and self-regulation. Any student can be a leader if they are happy to!

ADVANCING SKILLS: SUPPORTING AWARENESS OF METER, ACCENT AND STRESS

The above activities focus mainly on teaching durational contrasts in rhythm, but we also can use songs, rhymes and rhythm activities to emphasize the more subtle acoustic qualities of speech. The subtle changes in sound that make musical meter, for example, are critical for our developing skills in language perception (see Chapter 3). We can use sound and movement to promote awareness of metrical accents. When playing, saying or clapping rhythms, you can make the first word/syllable in each bar louder to draw attention to the metrical accent; and if you are also using actions, you could make the action larger. We can encourage the embodiment of metrical accent by asking learners to stamp the strong beat, so they begin to hear and feel the change: as we saw in Chapter 2, the ways we move or are moved to music help us to 'hear' meter. You can use sounds to teach this, too. For example, you can demonstrate a stronger accent by playing the strong beat on a physically larger instrument than the weaker beats, or on an instrument that has a different tone or more resonance.

We can simultaneously develop metrical awareness through sound, vision and movement when we play games and songs. For example, the Kodály play-song 'Bounce High, Bounce Low' (notation, game instructions and audio file are available at the Kodály Center – see 'Recommended resources' at the end of this chapter) uses actions that show the meaning of the words. The game's object is to bounce a ball between partners or members of a group, timing the ball's bounce to coincide with the downbeat. The sound of the ball as it bounces and its visual rhythm emphasize the strong beat, making it more salient. As with many Kodály songs, the lyrics can be easily personalized: my students used the game to learn and say each other's names – doing this often disrupted the game's rhythm, but it enabled the activity to be used for social interaction and vocalizing, as well as for developing rhythm awareness and motor coordination, and the ability to speak another's name rhythmically. Once the song is learned through the game, Kodály rhythm syllables can be used to teach rhythms of words or phrases, with or without the stick notation. This can be used as a priming activity to support the perception of the rhythm of the words or phrase before you ask the learner to speak the phrase rhythmically.

Ta Ta **Ta** Ta **Tee**-tee Tee-tee (**Ta**-Ta)

Bounce high, **bounce** low; **bounce** the ball to (**Shi**-loh)

Example: A group activity to develop rhythmic perception and bodily motor movement

While an external rhythm alone can support motor movement and gait, we can also consider using songs, chants and singing games. For example, the song 'Snail' (in Houlahan & Tacka, 2015) accompanies an action game in which group members walk in a line and coil inwards, echoing the shape of a snail's shell. The game can be used to target multiple rhythm movements and to include learners who have different motor abilities and verbal abilities. For example, the activity can be more challenging by incorporating dual-motor activities, increasing the demands on fine motor skills and increasing attentional and conceptual processing demands (e.g. teaching music literacy). It can be made less challenging by focusing on movements to the pulse only, by altering the tempo (a little), by including modifications to support motor movement (such as modified beaters, head nodding, blinking) and by supporting perception with additional auditory visual cues, such as puppets, notation or bells on feet. For example:

- Level 1: walk to the pulse – set the pace and beat beforehand and walk in time as someone else sings; people who use wheelchairs could use large motor movements to show the pulse.
- Level 2: walk to the rhythm of the words – set the pace, take large steps for the word snail (worth a count of one beat); take small quick steps to the words 'round and round and round we go' (each word is half a beat). People who use wheelchairs can use smaller limb movements to show the rhythm.
- Level 3: walk/move to the pulse and sing the words (if verbal).
- Level 3: walk/move to the pulse and simultaneously clap/flap/tap the words.

Further adaptations:

- Perform any of these activities as a 'round' – have two groups singing the song while walking the pulse.
- When seated, ask group members to 'show' the rhythm of the words as they sing or listen to a leader sing the song.
- Ask them to differentiate between pulse and rhythm; for example, stamp the pulse, clap the rhythm, tap alternate knees or shoulders to show the pulse, tap fingers or claves to show the rhythm.
- Use props – bounce a ball to the pulse while singing/listening; use hand puppets to 'nod' their head to the pulse or mouth the words.
- Continue with music literacy (see Chapter 2 – Find the heartbeat of a song) and attach rhythm names and symbols to the words. Over time, you can play the rhythm with instruments, read the music and play it backwards, and begin to attach melody. (See Video 5 in the online resources for an example.)

Using rhythm syllables (vocables)

Drum rhythm syllables (vocables) can make accented beats more tangible. Drum syllables are used for different purposes in drumming circles; they can emulate the sounds of the drum, or they can imitate the sound of the voice – we explored this idea in Chapter 3 when we looked at how the Bora people were able to use drums as a substitute for speech. Both purposes help support rhythm for speech. For example, suppose we transform a spoken phrase or song into Kodály rhythms (such as the *ta*, and *tee* in 'Bounce High, Bounce Low'). In that case, we can more easily draw attention to the duration of the words. Additionally, the rhythm can be easier to process in this way. The rhythm syllables are nonsensical and are vocally simple, and as a result, they do not require semantic processing or phonological processes.

However, we can use drum syllables for more than teaching rhythmic duration. Drum syllables capture the pitch and timbre of different beats as they are played on a drum. They can teach rhythmic sequences but also help young people to pay attention to tone and dynamics and explore and practise various limb-motor movements. For example, in the West African tradition of djembe, the vocables demonstrate rhythm sequences and guide actions: 'gun/dun' or 'bass' is an instruction to play in the centre of the drum, producing a 'deep' sound; 'go/do' or 'tone' is placed towards the edge of the drum, where it makes a medium-pitched tone; and 'ga/da' or 'slap' is a higher-pitched tone that is created by sharply slapping the rim with less of the palm and fingers making contact (see Video 10 in the online resources for an example). If we encourage learners to hear and make these simple, contrasting sounds, we can help them listen for the same types of acoustic changes that signal accent, meter and stress.

Sound poems: supporting word rhythm, meaning and creativity

Poems and rhymes can be used to support the ability to perceive and understand the rhythms of language. You can use poems or rhymes to draw attention to different layers of rhythm, from single sounds to syllable patterns and rhyme to stress and accent (see Chapter 6). For example, you can use a poem to develop attention to durational contrasts within words, patterning or syllables across a phrase, and stress accents of single words or whole phrases and rhyme. A 'sound poem' can be used as a basis of a rhythm poem: sound poems exploit and play with the sound of words or use onomatopoeic words. These can help children and young people explore sound creatively and examine the meaning of words; you can also ask children and young people to create their sound poems.

In her book, *Constructing Musical Healing*, June Boyce-Tillman (2000, p.286) gives an example of using her poem *Winter Solstice* to support a sense of connection between group members. Here is the first verse of her poem:

> The earth freezes;
> The crystals sparkle in the red sinking sun;
> The trees are bare;
> The shadows slant in a blackness the soft light cannot dispel.

Boyce-Tillman uses the piece to explore imagery and a sense of wonder in people who do not have language differences. You might be able to use her poem in this way, too. However, there are multiple ways to use such a poem for developing verbal skills. You can allocate specific lines to individuals or small groups in a group setting. They can find and create sounds to represent the meaning of a word or phrase; they can play the sound on cue as you recite the poem; they can silently read and play their part; you could cue them to play their sound in turn. Playing the rhythm of the words will give a very different feel to this poem. In this context, you might take the rhythm of one line (e.g. 'the trees are bare') and layer the sounds related to meaning on top of this. The differences in rhythm between lines one and three are subtle, and tasks like this can help you draw attention to word stress while giving the learners creative control and room to explore their musicality.

CHAPTER SUMMARY

For all children and young people – even those who are not yet verbal – rhythmic musical activities can be used to support a range of skills that underpin speech perception and production. Even simple rhythmic movement and rhythmic priming activities, such as playing a word's rhythm when cued, can involve different cognitive, physical and perceptual skills. We can use rhythmic games to target specific verbal skills, too, from elementary levels (such as attending to durational contrasts or turn-taking cues) to more advanced skills, such as layering word-based rhythms to create, and track, complex patterns; or to support awareness and control of accent and meter. As we saw in the examples of drumming and percussion activities earlier, and the *Winter Solstice* sound poem, we can use a single musical activity to practise more than one skill. If you work alongside professionals such as speech and language therapists, occupational therapists, music therapists and physiotherapists, you can use any type of rhythmic music game to support multiple skills. At the same time, learners will have fun and develop their musical abilities.

RECOMMENDED RESOURCES – RHYTHM GAMES AND ACTIVITIES

Abramson, R.M. (1997). *Feel It! Rhythm Games for All*. Book and CD. Miami, FL: Warner Brothers.

Berger, D.S. (2015). *Eurhythmics for Autism and Other Neurophysiologic Diagnoses: A Sensorimotor Music-Based Treatment Approach*. London: Jessica Kingsley Publishers.

'Bounce High, Bounce Low'. Kodály Center for Music Education: https://kodaly.hnu.edu/song.cfm?id=854.

Dworsky, A. (2013). *Slap Happy: How to Play World-Beat Rhythms with Just Your Body and a Buddy*. Santa Ynez, CA: Dancing Hands Music.

Faulkner, S. (2016). *Rhythm to Recovery: A Practical Guide to Using Rhythmic Music, Voice and Movement for Social and Emotional Development*. London: Jessica Kingsley Publishers.

Masala, K.S. & Presence, C. (2004). *Rhythm Play! Rhythm Activities and Initiatives for Adults, Facilitators, Teachers, & Kids!* Denver, CO: FUNdoing Publications.

PART 2

Vocal Skills

CHAPTER 6

The Foundations of Voice: Breathing and Posture

THE BIG QUESTIONS

What types of difficulties can young people have with breathing and posture, and how do these affect their voice? How can I support them to breathe when speaking, playing instruments or singing?

By the end of this chapter, you will:

- understand the relationships between breathing, posture and voice
- know why some groups of people have difficulties in controlling posture and breathing
- know some ideas that you can try to help young people develop easier, deeper breathing and respiratory capacity and strength.

WHO IS THIS FOR?

The information and ideas in this chapter can apply to all children and young people and will support skills in breathing for singing and speech. However, the chapter is especially relevant for those who have physiological or neurological differences that affect breathing and posture. These include people with *cerebral palsy, Down syndrome, hypermobility spectrum disorders, dyspraxia* and people with *sensory processing or integration difficulties*, especially proprioceptive difficulties that can occur in *hypermobility spectrum disorder (HSD)/hypermobile Ehlers Danlos syndrome (h-EDS), dyspraxia, autism* and *ADHD*.

Case study: Sammy

Sammy loved to sing. He sang with infectious enthusiasm and joy, adding dramatic poses and gestures as he performed to anyone who would watch him. His pleasure was clear, but so too was the stress his body was under as he aimed to reach and sustain long notes: he was determined not to take a breath until the end of the phrase.

Like so many young people I worked with, Sammy found it difficult to manage breathing for voice work. I remember him most clearly, though, because he was in my first singing group: I had never taught before and was anxious to get it right. I had read some 'how to teach kids to sing' books and chose some classic exercises to help him. I made sure to adapt them, so they were as tangible as possible – so that Sammy could feel and see that he was doing it right, as could I.

'Sammy, lie on the floor, please.'

'OK.'

'Now,' I said, 'I am going to place this book on your belly. Is that OK?'

'OK.'

'Now the book is on your belly, can you feel it?'

'Yes, I can.'

'OK, so I want you to take a deep breath and make the book move up in the air.'

Sammy did as I asked. The book rose as he pressed his shoulders into the floor, arched his back and raised his hips. Hm. Not quite what I expected. Over the next few sessions, I tried other approaches: 'Sammy, put this belt around your waist. Can you feel it? Can you breathe in so the belt moves out and gets tighter?' Sammy obliged, pushing down to make his waist expand. I tried again, 'OK, take a big breath and blow this pinwheel'; 'take a breath and blow this whistle'; 'watch me, Sammy...now copy me'. Each time, Sammy tensed part of his body, lifted his shoulders to breathe in, pushed out his belly and brought tension and stress.

What was going wrong? Were my instructions unclear? Did Sammy not understand? I discussed my observations with his speech and language therapist. 'That sounds like dyspraxia,' she said. She explained that this meant that there was not always clear communication between the brain and the muscles, so that a person might have difficulty in making some movements, even if they wanted to. That seemed to make sense, but left me with a problem: how to help

> Sammy develop his breathing so he could sing more easily, without putting his voice under such stress.

Over the years since Sammy, I have worked with many other young people whose natural response to 'take a breath' is to brace themselves. At its worst, this involves shoulders lifted, chest out, belly tight, throat closed, all of which restrict the movements needed for relaxed, deep breathing, and inhibit voice production. I only really began to find some answers to this as I embarked on my PhD and began to untangle some of the physiological, sensory and cognitive elements that affected how people like Sammy apply their breath to their voice. We will look at some of these issues in more detail in forthcoming chapters; but the starting point is with the body. If we can help our learners find their optimum posture for breathing and become more aware of their movements, we can better support them for using their voice.

This chapter will discuss some of the factors that can affect breath and posture in children and young people with physiological and sensory differences. We begin the chapter with an overview of the basic functions of breathing, so that it is easier to understand what is involved when singing or speaking. Next, with support from physiotherapist Tracey Gjertsen, we look at how posture affects our full breathing potential and, consequently, our voice. We then consider how posture and positioning affect breathing in learners with sensory and physical differences to understand better what adaptations we might make. Tracey provides some advice on developing posture for breathing when seated (Video 8) and standing (Video 9) (you can access her videos in the online resources). Finally, there are ideas to support breathing for voice, using song-based activities and musical instruments. However, I recommend that you work alongside a physiotherapist for any child or young person who exhibits chronic postural problems. Even quite subtle postural differences can have significant consequences.

BREATH, POSTURE AND VOICE

The act of breathing involves the movement of bodily systems that stretch from our nose to our abdomen (Titze & Martin, 1994; Sataloff, 2017). As we will see, the whole of our body can affect how well we breathe, but the primary organs are situated within the lower respiratory tract. The lower respiratory tract consists of the larynx, trachea, bronchi and lungs (see Figure 6.1). When we breathe in, air passes through our nose and pharynx (the upper respiratory tract) to our larynx. The larynx contains our vocal folds, which are situated above the trachea (windpipe), a cartilaginous tube that extends into the throat. We can use our vocal folds to seal the airway: we might do this when we hold our breath, for example. The larynx is positioned in front of the oesophagus, which leads to our stomach: our epiglottis at the top of the larynx spans both tubes and can act as a valve to seal off the airway into the trachea, for example to prevent food entering the airway. The base of the trachea splits into two airways (bronchi) which enter the left and right lung. Each bronchus then splits into smaller bronchioles, which fill each lung with increasingly smaller branches, like an inverted tree. Each bronchiole ends with a small enclosed sac (alveolus) that expands with air as we breathe in, transfers oxygen to the blood and expels carbon dioxide as we breathe out. These structures give our lungs a 'spongy' texture.

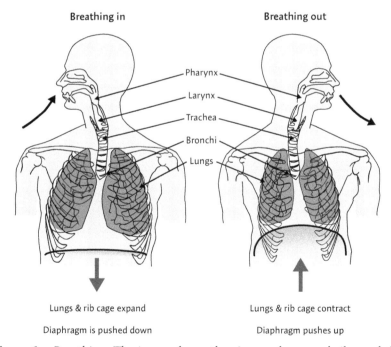

Figure 6.1: Breathing. The image shows the airways, lungs and ribs, and the movement of the ribs and diaphragm during breathing. The ribs expand and the diaphragm descends on inhalation; the ribs contract and the diaphragm ascends on exhalation.

The lungs sit within the rib cage, on either side of the heart. They are joined to the rib cage via two pleural membranes and are separated from the abdomen by the diaphragm, an elastic membrane made of muscle and connective tissue. Physiotherapist Tracey Gjertsen explains which organs and muscles are involved in breathing, and why posture is so important for efficient breathing:

> The diaphragm's efficiency relies on its mechanical attachment to the rib cage and fascial connections with the pelvic floor, neck and jaw. The area of attachment between the diaphragm and the rib cage – the zone of apposition – relies on abdominal muscle function, and on posture. In sub-optimal posture the diaphragm reaches a lower point of tension and has a reduced ability to draw air into the lungs. Optimal seated and standing stability requires the coordination of various muscles: the transverse abdominus, multifidus, internal obliques, pelvic floor and diaphragm. Co-contraction (simultaneous activity across muscle groups) increases intra-abdominal pressure and creates stiffness and stability in the lumbar spine. This allows the full excursion of the diaphragm by maintaining the zone of apposition. Deep abdominal muscle training can help improve trunk stability and respiratory function and is essential for the effective production of maximum inspiratory (MIP) and expiratory pressures (MEP).

When we consider that breathing involves connections that span from our jaw to our pelvis, we can understand why posture is crucial for breathing. As Tracey goes on to explain, the position and movement of our spine, sternum and rib cage are also critical:

> To draw air into the lungs, thoracic volume must increase, first by the downward movement of the diaphragm and second by increasing the diameter of the thoracic cage. The sternum moves upwards and outwards, and the rib cage expands sideways and upwards (see Figure 6.1). These movements are known as the pump handle and bucket handle mechanisms, and both are reliant on and limited by movement of the thoracic vertebrae.

We do not usually need to take conscious control of our breathing. Breathing usually comes under the control of our most primitive brain areas. As Tracey explains: 'The respiratory centres in the brain respond to oxygen and carbon dioxide levels in the blood; they trigger changes in respiration and ventilation rates to maintain a delicate balance'. However, we sometimes need to actively control breathing when *singing*, *speaking* or playing *wind instruments*. In passive breathing, the various expiratory muscles can simply relax as we breathe out, but in controlled breathing, we need to hold them contracted for longer and let them relax slowly and smoothly. In singing, this may be referred to as breath control, breath management or support. As Tracey explained, this control stems from our abdominal muscles as well as from the muscles of our upper chest. Whether we are seated or standing, good breathing, and controlled breathing, begin with postural control.

Postural problems, breathing and voice
While many of us find it easy to speak from any physical position, we will have greater difficulty using our voice if we have poor physical alignment – especially if poor posture becomes a habit. If we look at the physical processes involved in breathing and voice production from the head downwards, we can see how easily voice production can be disrupted. For example, someone who sits or walks with a forward head position will send their whole body out of alignment: a forward head creates tension at the back of the neck, and elongates the muscles of the upper spine; the muscles at the front of the thoracic cage will be contracted, and the space for lungs to expand will be reduced. Tracey explains how poor postural habits limit our breathing capacity:

> Upright sitting postures recruit greater activity in the pelvic floor muscles and internal obliques than slumped sitting (Sapsford *et al.*, 2008). Albarrati *et al.*, (2018) found that slouched sitting reduced respiratory muscle strength. They postulated that restriction of the rib cage in slouched sitting alters the articulations between the thoracic vertebrae and ribs and limits the contractility of the diaphragm. Other studies have reported reduced respiratory capacity and increased respiratory effort in slouched sitting. They suggest that slouching alters the length-tension relationship of the inspiratory muscles, reducing the functional capacity of the diaphragm.

Sitting with poor posture will reduce how we breathe for voice; but standing and moving with poor posture are also deleterious. One of the first people to make a connection between posture and voice was Frederick Matthias Alexander (1869–1955), founder of the Alexander Technique. He began to observe and experiment with his own posture when he experienced throat problems when reciting Shakespeare (Nicholls, 2014). The problems were alleviated by voice rest, but inflammation returned as soon as he began to recite again. Using a mirror, he observed that as he prepared to speak, he pulled his head backwards, lifted his chest, arched his spine and stiffened his legs – thereby creating tension and imbalance from his head to his toes. He concluded that this had direct consequences for his voice because his neck position altered the delicate balance of muscles within his throat that were responsible for producing voice. Additionally, his altered head position limited the movement of his ribs and diaphragm, and therefore, his lungs.

Since Alexander's experiment on himself, research evidence confirms that even minor alterations in the body can affect the production of voice. An entire chapter is dedicated to the effects of poor posture on voice in the book *Treatment of Voice Disorders* (Sataloff, 2017). The author stresses that the effects of even minor postural changes are significant for singing. Small postural changes may also be important for speech. This is such a critical issue that the effects of posture on muscles of the upper airways and larynx will be examined in greater detail in Chapter 7. For now, it is sufficient to recognize that:

- there is a relationship between how the whole body moves and how voice is ultimately produced
- some people are at risk of postural problems that can interfere with the efficient breathing needed for phonation
- supporting the whole body can improve breathing and voice.

POSTURE, VOICE AND BREATHING IN SPECIFIC NEEDS
We turn now to examine in more detail how posture and voice can lead to vocal problems in people who have physiological or sensory needs. The sections below illustrate the different ways in which breathing can be affected; their aim is to highlight symptoms you can look out for and to help you identify what adaptations you can easily and safely make and whether you need additional advice.

Breathing and postural difficulties in hypermobility disorders

Cat: posture, voice and hypermobility

Cat was an amateur singer who was experiencing intermittent voice loss. There was no sign of inflammation or irritation, but her voice would sometimes just stop or get stuck. After an ear, nose and throat (ENT) evaluation showed nothing that could explain her symptoms, a doctor suggested she went for professional voice coaching.

Cat found a vocal coach who specialized in voice problems in professional, performing opera singers. Ed, her coach, was in his seventies and had been fixing voice problems for decades. When he met Cat, he was struck by how quiet and weak her voice seemed when talking, and about how much effort she would put into 'trying' to make her voice ring with the 'buzz' that it should. Sometimes, almost by accident, she would find that buzz and her voice would flow freely and with the volume required for unamplified performance. These moments were rare, but gave him insight into her voice; her voice itself, as the ENT specialists had observed, was fine.

Ed was familiar with Alexander Technique and he noticed that several habits of Cat were likely to limit her voice. First, she tried too hard: this created anxiety and tension throughout her body, but especially in her throat. Second, her breathing was shallow and tight, with limited movement to the upper portion of her ribs. She also stood with knees locked and back arched. Until she learned to correct these habits, her voice would also remain locked. As an experiment, Ed asked Cat to try out different positions for singing – sitting, lying down in foetal position. Some inhibited the voice, some freed the voice; but all changed it. For Cat, overcoming these habits took years: exacerbated by a hypermobility spectrum disorder (HSD) which resulted in weaker postural muscles, as well as difficulties with prolonged standing, and frequent throat infections. However, she paid patient attention to developing and correcting the whole-body habits that created tension, and eventually found how to produce a resonant, easy voice for both speaking and singing.

As we see in Cat's story, someone can have difficulties breathing for voice because of their posture, physiology and emotional state. Children and young people who are hypermobile may have musculoskeletal differences that affect how they breathe. These could include atypical curvature of the spine (e.g. scoliosis), weak intercostal muscles, or ribs that sublux (partially dislocate) (Castori *et al.*, 2010; Castori 2012). Some can experience 'floppiness' in their airways, leading to asthma-like symptoms as the tissues of the airways collapse inwards and cause partial obstruction or narrowing. This can cause wheezing and difficulties breathing (Morgan *et al.*, 2007; Harris *et al.*, 2013). These types of physiological problems can lead to pain or discomfort, and also distress. The 'collapse' of airways and feeling of being unable to fully breathe in can be frightening and its emotional impact can disrupt breathing further.

Changes to breathing may also occur in people with hypermobility who also have dysautonomia or postural orthostatic tachycardia syndrome (POTS) – an upright position can affect blood flow and heart rate, which can cause palpitations, feelings of dizziness or fainting, and feelings of stress and anxiety (Fedorowski, 2018). These feelings of stress can stiffen the diaphragm and affect breathing and lead to symptoms similar to those of a panic attack. These complex interactions can make it hard for people with hypermobility to breathe fully and control airflow for speech and for singing.

The effects of hypermobility are individual and complex. To support breathing for speech, song or playing musical instruments, the primary focus should be on supporting posture and relaxed muscles during the in-breath, and on developing muscular control during the out-breath to stop the posture and lungs collapsing. However, people with HSD or h-EDS who have vulnerable joints within the respiratory system may be at risk of injury through over-use, or through subluxations, which are often unpredictable. It is therefore important to keep exercises that involve movement within safe limits. Additionally, exercise may trigger feelings of breathlessness and asthma-like symptoms during or after exercise and feelings of chronic fatigue. People with hypermobility may need a careful programme of physiotherapy to help them develop muscle strength; this will help stabilize vulnerable joints, thereby reducing the risk of injury, and will support posture. They may also need mobility aids and splints to support them when they experience a flare-up of symptoms.

Careful observation will be needed to support the child or young person with hypermobility: reduced proprioception and increased sensations of pain may make it more difficult for them to identify habits that affect the efficiency of their breathing. For example, they may not be aware of muscle tension in the head or shoulders, or of over-extended knees; they may habitually hold a 'forward-head' position; they may hold tension in their abdomen. Each of these will reduce the ability to breathe efficiently. Furthermore, these symptoms may fluctuate or change over time as a result of injury (e.g. subluxation, over-stretching), joint pain, and muscle stiffness, pain, fatigue and hormonal changes. For females, changes in the hormones progesterone and oestrogen can lead to worsening of some symptoms (Graf *et al.*, 2019), such as an increase in laxity and joint dislocations. It may be helpful for you to use a diary to track any cyclical changes, or to encourage the young person or their carer to monitor these.

Breathing and postural differences in Down syndrome

Someone with Down syndrome can have difficulty breathing because of *anatomical differences*, *hypermobility*, and poor levels of *health and fitness*. Many people with Down syndrome have lungs that develop with a lower number of alveoli and bronchiole, reducing the surface area available for expansion and gas exchange. They may also develop differences in anatomy and soft tissue in the upper airways. In particular, the cartilage in the larynx, trachea and bronchi is often reported as soft or floppy (Bertrand *et al.*, 2003). Where such floppiness occurs in the larynx (laryngomalacia), the larynx above the vocal folds can partially obstruct the airways. Where this softness occurs in the trachea (tracheomalacia) or bronchial tubes (bronchomalacia) the airways may partially collapse, restricting breathing, and producing wheezing. Many people with Down syndrome also have narrower airways, with further narrowing reported below the vocal folds and above the trachea (see Pandit & Fitzgerald, 2012 for a review).

Breathing in people with Down syndrome may also be affected by weaknesses in the muscles that drive and support respiration. For example, if a child has weak muscles that open the ribs during inhalation, they may have smaller chest expansion. The primary cause of these weaknesses stems from lax ligaments and reduced muscle tone, but people with Down syndrome often also have increased weight and inactive lifestyles, which can exacerbate any muscular weaknesses. Unfortunately, this effect is circular: muscle weakness and hypermobility make exercise much harder and can produce unpleasant symptoms, including feelings of breathlessness, fatigue and weakness (Soyucen & Esen, 2010); but lack of exercise and increasing weight can make it harder for them to increase muscle tone and reduce symptoms. People with Down syndrome are already at risk of having reduced oxygen intake and energy because of weak respiratory muscles and low airflow. Additionally, they may have conditions that disrupt their sleep, such as sleep apnea, and altered breathing patterns (Dumortier & Bricout, 2020). These health conditions can make exercise challenging as they can reduce energy and affect attention, learning and cardiovascular function.

In addition to the effects of altered lung function, people with Down syndrome typically have difficulties in maintaining a stable, balanced posture. In part, this may be due to their anatomy, muscle differences and lax ligaments. Typically, unless corrected, someone with Down syndrome is likely to move with an altered head position, may over-extend their lower back, lock or turn their knees inwards, and have flat arches and inward-rolling ankles. In addition, they may have curvature of the spine, instability of the neck, low muscle tone, motor coordination difficulties, motor timing difficulties that make them slower to react, poor proprioception, difficulties in maintaining balance, and frequent upper respiratory tract infections. Any of these conditions can negatively impact a breathing system that is already compromised.

While it is not possible to address every factor that can affect breathing, research has shown that people with Down syndrome become better at motor movements with appropriate teaching and practice. Over time, careful, structured support for movement and muscle development can successfully reduce the effects of poor postural habits and strengthen muscles and posture (Georgiadis *et al.*, 2019). Meanwhile, it may be helpful to find alternative ways to support breathing for singing: as for Cat, supine postures might release tension in the muscles and reduce strain for voice work – but be mindful of Sammy, who used extra effort to breathe in this position! Physical splints or corsets might increase proprioceptive feedback and provide support while developing awareness and control of breathing.

Breathing differences in autism and other sensory needs

Breathing differences have been identified in some people with autism and with ADHD (Ming *et al.*, 2016). In comparison to people without autism or ADHD, they are more likely to have differences in lung function and are also at increased risk of developing respiratory disorders. Some children and young adults in these groups are also more likely to breathe through their mouth, rather than through their nose. Mouth-breathing can change the quality of breathing and cause dryness, which can negatively affect voice production. In people with autism, at-rest breathing patterns may be less smooth and regular than in people without autism. Some people with autism may breathe faster than people without autism; their breathing may also be shallower and they may hold their breath. The cause is linked to *autonomic dysfunction*, which can lead to under- or over-arousal in the central nervous system. These altered styles of breathing can affect the parasympathetic nervous system which helps us regulate emotions. As a result, this style of breathing might contribute to higher anxiety and hypervigilance, which can be common in people with autism.

A sub-group of people with neurodevelopmental disorders such as *ADHD*, *Tourette's* and *autism* are at increased risk of hypermobility, which can also increase stress response because of autonomic differences, and reduce muscle tone or strength, affecting respiration. It is possible that the breathing differences observed in people with these needs can contribute to anxiety and result from physiological differences that exacerbate symptoms of anxiety and panic attacks. In both cases, supporting deeper breathing and slower exhalations can help calm the nervous system and reduce symptoms of anxiety and stress. As with hypermobile groups, there is also evidence that posture and proprioception are altered in some children and young people with autism. They may have greater difficulties than their peers in maintaining balance due to difficulties in integrating the information they receive from their different senses – including vision, touch, and their sense of balance. Similarly, some people with *autism*, *ADHD* and *dyspraxia* might have altered breathing patterns as a result of sensory processing differences. Difficulties in volitional motor control and breathing can both occur in people with dyspraxia – Sammy in the case study represents a real but possibly extreme example of how altered proprioception may affect an ability to deliberately control breathing.

HOW DO I BEGIN TO SUPPORT BREATHING FOR VOICE?

Breathing exercises are an essential part of training for singing and offer many additional benefits for energy, health and wellbeing. Suitable exercises can improve the strength and function of respiratory muscles. However, the first process of supporting breathing is to identify whether and how breathing is affected by posture, underlying health conditions, autonomic disorders and muscular weaknesses. You can then build posture-strengthening activities and breathwork into musical activities to help children and young people develop awareness and control of their breathing. This is the first step towards developing a healthy voice, as we will see in Chapter 7.

Observe posture

We can use observation to understand the effects of these needs on a learner's posture and breathing. It may be helpful to observe multiple times to understand why they have difficulty in producing or using their voice. For example, consider how they breathe when seated and when standing and how they hold their body when static and moving. The goal for observations should be to recognize possible complicating factors – not necessarily to correct them, but to identify contributing factors and priorities for immediate support, and to establish if there is a 'best' form of posture for breathwork.

POSTURAL POSITION

The optimal shape of the spine in standing will demonstrate four distinct curves: the cervical and lumbar lordoses and the thoracic and sacral kyphoses, with the pelvis held in a 10–15-degree anterior tilt. A simple plumb line should pass through the ear lobe to the front of the ankle, traversing the heads of the humerus and femur and slightly anterior to the knee joint line (see Figure 6.2).

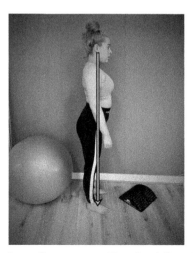

Figure 6.2: Optimal standing posture. The plumb line shows the optimal alignment from the ear to the front of the ankle.

Seated posture with the feet on the floor will demonstrate a slightly flattened lumbar lordosis and reduced anterior pelvic tilt to the neutral line.

Note how changes in spinal position affect head position (Figure 6.3).

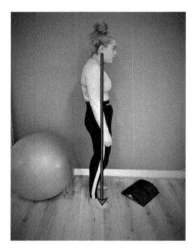 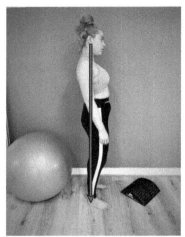

Figure 6.3: Altered spinal position with a) a forward-head position and b) a retracted head position. Notice how the plumb line moves from the optimal position as spinal position alters.

Optimal posture allows expansion of the rib cage in both transverse and sternal planes and extension in the upper thoracic region of the spine. These movements can be limited by posture-related stiffness in the thoracic spine. Prolonged slumped seated and standing habits can result in a stiff increased thoracic kyphosis and forward head posture where the accessory muscles pectoralis minor, sternocleidomastoid, scalenei and levator scapulae can become shortened and over-used. The accessory muscles provide assistance to the main muscles used for breathing and should be recruited to generate maximal inspiratory and expiratory force, not during restful breathing.

Exercises to strengthen the deep stabilizing muscles should be performed in both seated and standing positions before incorporating them into functional movement.

See Videos 8 and 9 in the online resources for exercises to support posture for breathing, in seated and standing positions.

Once the body is in its best position for breathing, there can be significant improvements for speech, even in children who have quite complex physical needs, such as cerebral palsy (Solomon & Charron, 1998). Even a few months of respiratory physiotherapy training by specialists can have significant effects for children with autism, ADHD and Down syndrome. In a study by Georgiadis and colleagues (2019), 56 children within these groups took part in respiratory physiotherapy for 30 minutes, three times a week for five months, while a control group took part in a programme of aerobic exercise. The children took part in relaxation exercises, controlled inhalation and exhalation, and respiratory training with specialist equipment; the programme also integrated breathing exercises using balloons, water and whistles. The results showed that the training led to improved oxygen levels in the bloodstream and a reduced heart rate. Furthermore, Tracey explains that specific inspiratory muscle training in children with Down syndrome and cerebral palsy has not only improved respiratory muscle strength but also trunk stability and exercise capacity, and that graded exercise programmes have been shown to improve postural strength, balance and function in populations with hypermobility and postural weakness.

Physical strengthening for breathing

Tracey Gjertsen gives some example activities, below, that you can use to develop and support the postural muscles. As with other exercises in the book, support from physiotherapists may be needed to ensure that the child is developing healthy postural and muscular habits. Specialist input will also ensure that children are benefitting fully from activities.

SUPPORTING POSTURAL MUSCLE: SUGGESTED EXERCISES FROM TRACEY GJERTSEN

Seated (see also Video 8)

To find the neutral position in seated, begin with the feet flat on the floor at hip width. There should be equal pressure felt through each sit bone.

Try to sit back into the pelvis onto the sacrum (lumbar flexion) and then roll forwards to bring more weight into the pubic bone (lumbar extension). Now find your mid-point where your sit bones are the central point and the pelvis is in neutral.

Place your hand just over the navel and draw the tummy

muscles in to pull the navel slightly away from your hand – hold for ten seconds and breathe normally. Repeat ten times.

When you have mastered this, add some arm or leg movement.

Find your neutral sitting position; draw the abdominal muscles in as before. Slowly raise the right arm without leaning back or allowing the shoulder to lift up towards the ear. Repeat this five times with each arm.

This exercise can be repeated lifting the foot away from the floor without twisting the pelvis backwards or leaning over.

Standing (see also Video 9)

To find your neutral position, stand with your feet at hip width, place your hand on your sternum (breastbone.) Now lift your sternum up into your hand; notice how this changes your head and lumbar spine into a more extended position. Drop the sternum into a flexed or stooped position; again notice the changes in your head and lumbar spine position. Find your mid-point when the head is sitting directly over your shoulders (Figure 6.2).

Now place your hands on top of the pelvis and tilt the pelvis backwards – imagine that if this were a bucket of water you are now spilling water towards your heels – and forwards, so that water spills onto your toes. Find the point where no water would spill out of your bucket – this is neutral.

Draw the abdominal muscles in as before and hold for ten seconds while breathing normally. Repeat ten times.

When you have mastered this, you can add some arm and leg movement as before.

Supporting breathing for singing and music

Books in the 'Recommended reading' section provide many exercises to try, but below are a few that are effective for developing awareness and control of the muscles, and that can be incorporated easily into singing or music-based sessions, where they can become part of everyday musical play or practice. These activities focus on inhalation, exhalation and breathing with movement. The exercises incorporate multisensory stimuli, where possible, to encourage children and young people to see, hear and feel the movement – this is especially important if they have poor proprioception or other sensory differences. Given that some children may have sensory sensitivities or physical vulnerabilities, though, adjust any exercises to suit.

Exercises for inhalation

The aim of inhalation exercises is to develop awareness of breathing quickly for singing, speaking or playing an instrument without over-activating other muscles in the body, such as we saw in the example of Sammy. These are designed to develop good habits for singing and voice, but may also support aspects of wellbeing by encouraging slower and deeper forms of breathing. If needed, make activities multisensory – this can help develop awareness when some senses, such as proprioception or interoception, are weak. In all activities, aim to focus on maintaining good postural alignment, especially in the head, neck and shoulders.

'Sniff a flower' (or other scented object). A sniff tends to open the lower ribs outwards without excessive force or tension arising in the upper chest, neck or shoulders. Begin with anything that smells good (flowers, candles, chocolate) and practise taking a long, deep sniff, and then short sequences of small sniffs. You could follow with a slow, relaxed sigh as we move into connecting breath and voice.

Use a harmonica/mouth organ. Breathing in through a harmonica makes the in-breath audible, as well as the out-breath. This provides useful auditory cues about the quality of the in-breath: is it smooth and relaxed, or jagged and 'forced' in sound?

Sip slowly through a straw. This can reduce the tendency to breathe into the upper chest, promoting deeper breathing without tension in the shoulders and elsewhere. Larger-bore straws can be used to assist with complete lip closure.

Exercises for exhalation

The focus of exhalation exercises is to develop the muscles that control air flow, while maintaining relaxed muscles in the upper body and neck, and good postural alignment. The main active muscles we use for controlling exhalation are those of the rib cage (the intercostal muscles) and the abdominal muscles: these help us control the rate of exhalation. If asked to sustain an out-breath, we may tend to 'collapse' the rib cage, or to introduce tension into the shoulders. Collapse occurs if we let the air out without control, allowing the ribs to be pulled downwards and to slump, and the spine to curve forward. The aim is to maintain a stable posture, while keeping the ribs open for as long as possible so that we use the intercostal muscles to gradually contract the ribs. For good control of the out-breath, there should be no change in the length or curvature of the spine: the ribs will close inwards but not downwards, and the abdominal muscles will tighten, without the body tilting forward. Depending on the volume of our vocalizations, we may feel our abdominal muscles move strongly (such as when we laugh) or more gently (such as when we sigh).

Activate the epigastrium. The epigastrium sits between the lower ribs and abdominal muscles and is one of the most important muscles for controlling exhalation. One of the easiest ways to feel this is to exhale while making a 'Tsss' sound.

Play wind instruments. Wind instruments require considerable sub-glottic force during playing. The force required to activate and maintain a steady note on a wind instrument (e.g. clarinet) is considerably higher than is required for singing. Theoretically, if you practise sustaining notes on a wind instrument, you will strengthen the breathing muscles that are required for controlled singing to a greater level than could be acquired through singing alone.

Blow whistles, recorders, melodicas. Bigger instruments and lower notes take more breath. These are excellent for developing breath control, but beware of rib collapse in extended notes! Aim to extend the quality of the sound, rather than duration. It may be easier to begin with high-pitched notes/instruments, as these require less breath for a good tone, although over-blowing can result in shrill notes and sudden pitch breaks. Recorders and whistles can also help develop muscles for lip closure – try different instruments, to find which sized mouthpieces best suit the child or person you work with.

Combining inhalation and exhalation with movement

Use visuals and a beat. You could make the coordination and timing of breathing multisensory by adding attractive visuals, such as coloured scarves or large scrunchie bands, and by moving in time to an audible beat. Visuals can be used to show and practise the movement and timing of breathing in and breathing out. For example, you can show slow breathing movements using coloured scarfs, or faster movements with a 'scrunchie' band. In pairs or small groups, inhale as the scarf or band goes up, and exhale as the scarf or band lowers. If working individually with scarves, you could combine this with a yoga-style movement, by lifting arms up slowly on the inhale and lowering them slowly on the exhale: this has the advantage of helping to open the ribs.

Many meditation apps or videos on the internet also have visual prompts for supporting breathing and for finding a rhythm in breathing: these are often a coloured circle that expands to a given count for breathing in, and shrinks to a beat for breathing out.

Blend movement, music and breath. You could create a simple movement routine to music that is based on a series of physical exercises designed to support and strengthen the rib cage and abdominal muscles, and promote relaxation. In his book, *Teaching Kids to Sing* (see 'Recommended resources'), Phillips gives a sequence of exercises that can be used to support awareness and control of breathing. However, some children and young people may have problems with maintaining posture and using correct muscle control when performing exercises, which could exacerbate problems. For some young people, you could use exercises from Pilates or Tai Chi to help build awareness and core strength at the beginning of music programmes, and to help wind down sessions. These activities include focused awareness on breathing, and have additional benefits for wellbeing. Yoga exercises may also be used but you may need to ensure that movements are controlled to avoid excessive reaching and stretching of the joints.

CHAPTER SUMMARY

Some of the young people we work with may have problems with breathing that arise from their unique physiological and sensory characteristics. To support their breathing for voice and music-making, we need to consider their whole body's positioning: even small disturbances in alignment can impede how much breath we can take, and how we control it for speaking, singing or playing instruments. People with physical and sensory differences can have difficulties in achieving the best posture for breathing: while it is important to strengthen posture for breathing, we also need to recognize that sometimes a compromise is needed. If maintaining an optimum position creates tension or physiological problems, it may be easier to try a new position that places less strain on the body. Alternatively, we might consider using mobility aids during exercises, with appropriate guidance or supervision. When developing breathing for voice work, we need to ensure that the in-breath is relaxed and that the out-breath is controlled. Multisensory teaching activities can help develop awareness and control of breathing. Musical instruments, especially wind instruments, can be useful in developing breath control, and provide audible cues about breath management and control. We can easily incorporate breathwork into a programme of wider music-based activities, but may need to observe carefully and adapt postures to ensure that the body is as free to move as possible, without strain.

RECOMMENDED READING

Dimon, T. (2018). *Anatomy of the Voice: An Illustrated Guide for Singers, Vocal Coaches, and Speech Therapists*. Berkeley, CA: North Atlantic Books.

Fisher, J. & Keyes, G. (2018). *This Is a Voice: 99 Exercises to Train, Project, and Harness the Power of Your Voice.* London: Wellcome Collection.

McCallion, M. (1998). *The Voice Book*. London: Faber & Faber.

Nicholls, C. (2014). *Body, Breath and Being: A New Guide to the Alexander Technique*. Hove: D&B Publishing.

Phillips, K. (2013). *Teaching Kids to Sing*. New York, NY: Schirmer.

CHAPTER 7

Producing Voice

THE BIG QUESTIONS

How do we produce our voice? How can I begin to support children and young people to use their voice more easily?

By the end of the chapter, you will:

- know how the laryngeal structures and our body work together to produce voice
- understand how and why problems in phonation and voice can occur
- know some general principles to support healthy voice function.

WHO IS THIS FOR?

This chapter is relevant to anyone who wishes to understand voice function and disorder, and how physical and psychological factors can lead to voice problems.

The ideas within are especially relevant to people who have difficulties in using their vocal folds, such as people with *cerebral palsy*, *Down syndrome*, *hypermobility spectrum disorders* (*HSD/h-EDS*), and those who are at risk of damaging their vocal folds through use, including people with *ADHD* and *autism*.

Case study: Amy

Amy is singing her favourite song. She is projecting well and hitting all the notes across her unusually large vocal range. Today, she seems to have good control: her breath management helps her sustain a lovely tone on sustained notes, across phrases; and to create subtle changes in volume. In full flow, she stops suddenly, coughing. 'What is it?' I ask. She looks at me, her face a mix of frustration, anger and pain, and gestures to her throat. 'Gone,' she whispers.

Our voices are robust instruments. A newborn baby can cry for hours and never damage the delicate membranes that create such impressive volume. But as we grow, some of us find our voice tires, hurts or breaks; like Amy, it might just stop mid-flow. What goes wrong? Usually, our body or our mind has interfered. As we saw in Chapter 6, a few adjustments to the whole body can sometimes fix the problem and set the voice free. However, our voice is deeply personal, and emotional factors like anxiety affect it as much as physiological or cognitive factors.

When we are working with children and young people who find it hard to use their voice, we need to consider how many factors could be involved, from the ground up. This chapter provides a basic understanding of how we produce voice. First, I introduce the anatomical properties of the vocal tract, and explain how we use our vocal folds to make sound, and our vocal tract to alter its quality. I build on Chapter 6, to show how our breathing and postural muscles enable us to produce voice. We then turn to voice disorder and I explain the main types of voice dysfunction, and look at how anxiety, hormonal and cognitive factors can affect voice. I will offer some general principles that can help you support young people to begin to use their voices without damaging them. In the next chapter, we will look more closely at voice difficulties in young people who have physiological, medical, sensory or cognitive differences that can interfere with voice.

HOW DO WE PRODUCE OUR VOICE?

Producing voice is a basic mechanical function that we share with birds and some other mammals, as well as with our earliest human ancestors. At its most basic, physical level, all we must do to produce rudimentary vocal communication is to force air to move in a continuous wave-like pattern (see Chapter 1). Consider, for example, the childhood games of holding a blade of grass between the thumbs and blowing, in order to produce a penetrating whistle. Or think of whistling: we can shape the oral cavity (tongue, soft palate, pharynx and lips) into several configurations that allow us to produce complex, melodic patterns made of air. Producing voice is so easy, it is the first thing we do after taking our first breath.

We do not have a dedicated mechanism that creates our voice: instead, our voice is assembled from parts of the body that evolved to do other jobs. These separate parts can move rapidly to form different configurations, enabling the vocal folds to shift in shape, size and length and to open and close against a pressurized column of air. These structures' speed, strength and flexibility make the voice incredibly adaptable in pitch, volume and tone. This endows singers and non-singers alike with an instrument that can produce hundreds of different sounds and a voice so unique it can act like a fingerprint. The following sections explain the physical processes that enable us to produce a vocal sound and alter its quality, and how we can sustain a vocal sound at a given pitch.

Vocal structures and phonation

Although the whole body influences our voice, the larynx is where the magic happens. The larynx is a cartilaginous structure that sits in the throat, atop the trachea, or windpipe. In adults, the larynx connects the pharynx (at the back of the mouth) to the trachea (at the top of the respiratory system). The trachea sits in front of the oesophagus, the muscly tube that joins our mouth to our stomach. Both tubes are topped by a leaf-shaped cartilage that connects like a hinge to the upper surface of the larynx. This cartilage, the epiglottis, opens during breathing, and closes when we swallow, protecting the airways from the accidental inhalation of food and drink. It can be challenging for us to feel the larynx as it moves, but you can feel or see the 'shield' cartilage that sits at the front of the neck, just under the jaw, visible in some as the Adam's apple (Figure 7.1). If we touch our fingers gently to this cartilage and make a vocal siren sound (up and down in pitch), we may feel the vibrations from the vocal folds within, and feel the larynx gently move up and down. If we swallow or cough, we will feel the movement more strongly.

The larynx is suspended within a delicately balanced web of muscles and ligaments, giving it mobility within the throat, and stability (see Figure 7.2; and see Dimon, 2018). Various muscles and ligaments help move and stabilize the larynx from above and below. Support from above comes from ligaments that attach the larynx to the horseshoe-shaped hyoid bone, which sits within the lower jaw and connects to the muscles of the tongue and pharynx, and to the jaw. The hyoid, and thereby the larynx which hangs from it, can be moved upwards by a group of muscles that attach to the jaw, the base of the skull and the soft palate muscles. These 'elevator' muscles can lift the larynx and exert slightly forwards and backwards forces. From below, the larynx is anchored by muscles extending from the hyoid bone to the sternum and towards the shoulders. The primary role of these muscles is for swallowing. When we swallow, the larynx ascends and the airway is covered by the epiglottis, protecting it from food. This vertical mobility plays an important role in voice control: the height of the larynx within the neck can be deliberately controlled by experienced singers to produce specific vocal effects and tones. However, the movement of the larynx may be constrained or altered if there is an imbalance in the muscles – that is, if one set is weak and another is strong. Unless we strengthen the weakened muscles that help move the larynx, we can develop voice problems (MaCallion, 1998; Dimon, 2018). This will be discussed in more detail in the sections below.

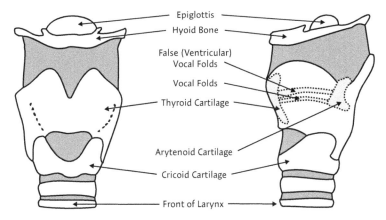

Figure 7.1: The larynx. This shows the external laryngeal structure: the thyroid cartilage is the bony part we can feel under our jaw – the Adam's apple. The vocal folds sit just behind this, spanning the airway, and connecting to the arytenoids.

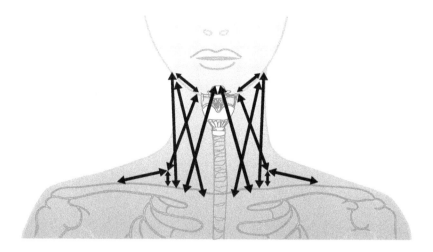

Figure 7.2: The larynx is anchored from above and below. The figure shows a simplistic representation of how various muscles give the larynx mobility and stability. The larynx is connected via muscles to the skull and the hyoid bone; and from below, it is anchored to the sternum and clavicle. These muscle groups need to be free to relax and contract so that the larynx is free to move. Altering the body's position can weaken, shorten or lengthen some of these stabilizing muscles, which can cause voice problems.

The shield-shaped thyroid cartilage at the front of the neck houses the vocal folds. The vocal folds are formed of mucous membrane that lines the larynx. The membrane forms two pairs of folds that jut into the space within the larynx. The upper pair form the false, or vestibular, vocal folds. These false vocal folds sit above the true vocal folds. When the vocal system is working optimally, the vocal folds are responsible for the act of phonation. However, as will be discussed later, some people may also deliberately engage the false (vestibular) vocal folds for specific effects, or accidentally.

The vocal folds are membranes 8–16 mm in length that stretch across the larynx, where they can close to seal the trachea. The vocal folds are made of layers with different physical properties. This enables them to change their size and function: they can increase in bulk, causing them to thicken; they can reduce in bulk, becoming thinner; they can lengthen or shorten; they can act something like a zipper – closing at the edge nearest the pharynx before, then 'zippering' to a close at their top edge (see Figure 7.3; and Video 6 in the online resources).

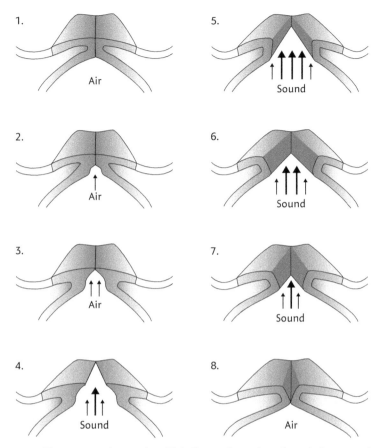

Figure 7.3: How we produce voice. This figure shows how breath from our lungs opens the vocal folds. When we want to speak or sing, the air in the trachea pushes against the closed vocal folds (1). As we increase the sub-glottal pressure, the air opens the different layers of the vocal folds gradually (2–4); at the same time, the folds open at their front first. This produces a 'zippering' effect. As the puff of air passes through the folds, the change in air pressure at the glottis 'sucks' the vocal folds closed and they zipper shut (5–8). Sound is produced as the vocal folds open and close. This opening and closing happens very quickly and creates the vocal 'buzz' that we can feel. (Figure is based on the work of Chen, 2016, and Hirano & Kakita, 1985.)

The edges of the vocal folds are supple, enabling them to vibrate at about 220 times per second for the average female. The rapid opening and closing of the vocal folds generate the audible 'buzz' of phonation. The regular movement of the vocal folds generates glottal pulses, known as *phonation*, or voicing. One cycle of abduction (opening) and adduction (closing) is the 'period' of the vibration: the number of periods produced per second is the *fundamental frequency* (F0: measured in hertz), which is perceived as 'pitch'. Several structures within the larynx contribute to changes in pitch, volume and perceived timbre of the voice. The thyroid cartilage is hinged, enabling it to tilt. This tilting action can affect pitch and volume as the movements alter the tension and length of the vocal folds. However, two key structures are the arytenoid cartilages which sit atop the thyroid cartilage at the front of the larynx: these pivot to open and close the vocal folds, creating a v-shaped glottal chink when fully open, closing the glottal chink fully (to seal the trachea), or partially closing the vocal folds to produce phonation (see Figure 7.4). The actions of these internal muscles, and the height of the larynx, affect the tension and thickness of the vocal folds; these actions contribute to the perceived pitch, loudness and quality of phonation. A general principle is that thin, stretched vocal folds create higher-pitched sounds, like a tensed guitar string. In contrast, shorter, thicker bulkier vocal folds create lower pitches and heavier, louder sounds. However, the final sound is also influenced by breath pressure and resonance.

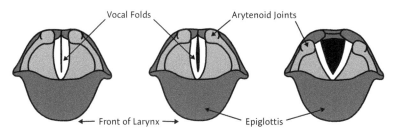

Figure 7.4: The opening of the vocal folds and movement of the arytenoids. The arytenoid joints are at the back of the larynx. They move to open the vocal folds.

TRY THIS AT HOME: BUILD YOUR OWN LARYNX

Jeremy Fisher of Vocal Process has created a free template that you can use to build your own model larynx. You can download the instructions from their website, and watch a YouTube video to show how to build it (see 'Recommended reading and resources'). You can play with the model to learn how the joints in the larynx fit together and move.

ACTIVATING THE VOICE: HOW DO WE SING A SINGLE VOWEL SOUND?

We might have a perfect vocal structure and fully functional muscles in our vocal tract, but there is no voice without breath. Breath is the energy source: its movement drives phonation and its speed and force carry the sound and contribute to its tone, and volume. However, we need just the breath pressure to produce phonation and this must be balanced by the right amount of tension in the vocal folds.

In preparation for singing a vocal sound – perhaps an /i/, as in 'sheep', at middle C – you must imagine the sound and pitch you wish to produce. As we saw in Chapter 3, hearing or imagining a movement can engage the muscles, anticipating the task ahead. In readiness to sing, the structures within your larynx move into position – the larynx remains low in the throat, the thyroid cartilage tilts slightly, adding tension to the vocal folds and altering the shape of the pharynx above the larynx. The soft palate lifts and the body of the tongue bunches up: this creates a shape within the vocal tract that lends the /i/ vowel its distinctive sound, and it simultaneously exerts a slight upwards and forwards pull on the larynx. To counteract this upwards/forwards movement, the sternum must lift and the shoulders must relax, stabilizing the larynx. The small muscles and arytenoids that alter the vocal fold mass and tension are poised to produce the desired pitch and tone, and the ear listens, ready to adjust the vocal muscles to maintain the desired sound and pitch.

Almost simultaneously, you breathe in. As you hold the air in the lungs and trachea, your intercostal muscles are fighting to keep the ribs open as they resist the inward pull of the forces for exhalation. At this point, we might close our vocal folds. In this state of balance, the air in the respiratory tract is held at constant pressure, but it is pushing outwards in all directions, including against the closed vocal folds. To stay closed, the vocal folds also exert a resistant force against the air pressure. You can feel this now: if you breathe in and suspend your breath for as long as you can and focus on where in your throat you are holding your breath, you will feel the muscles of your glottis actively resist the pressure from below.

Once we are ready to sing, we use small movements to push the pressurized air in our lungs against our vocal folds. To do this, our diaphragm can begin to rise to gently compress the air, increasing its pressure; or our lower ribs can move inwards, with the same effect. As the pressure builds, our breath forces the vocal folds to open: they open at the bottom, first, as the air pressure pushes against them. Next, the moving air pushes against and opens the top layer, and the bottom layers close. This creates a wave-like motion, rather than a simple opening and closing; and it allows the pressurized air to escape in little puffs.

A steady pitch and an effortless tone requires breath pressure that is *just enough* to initiate and sustain the wave-like oscillation of the vocal folds: too much or too little pressure may introduce strident or breathy tones, or accidentally change the frequency of vibration. When we sing an /i/ on middle C, with our tongue and larynx perfectly poised and the breath is 'just right', our vocal folds open and close at a rate of 256 cycles per second. We can then make subtle adjustments to the airflow, or the tension of the vocal folds to alter the sound and tone, without altering the rate at which the vocal folds oscillate. With everything just so, the energized, vibrating air meets our ears, and we perceive the vowel sound at the pitch we imagined.

Voice quality

In its raw form, the sound created by the oscillating vocal folds is mechanical – a sequence of rapid beeps, known as the glottal pulse (you can see an animated example of this in Video 6 in the online resources). The opening and closing of the vocal folds chops the air into segments resulting in a complex acoustic wave. The raw signal is unpleasant. It is enriched and transformed by our resonators: the larynx, pharynx, sinuses and upper chest. These spaces amplify the sound and add different tones. Like walls in rooms that soften sounds or create echoes, a harder or more tense structure will add brightness, whereas a softer surface might absorb and mute certain frequencies. As a result of the shape, size and physiological makeup of our resonators, the pulse becomes rich with overtones or harmonics, making our voices as individual and distinct as our fingerprints.

The vocal tract also helps us produce distinct vowels. It does this by adding certain types of harmonics to the raw sound. For example, when the tongue is raised in its middle towards the top of the hard palate, and the lips are open and slightly spread, the sound /i/ is produced (as in the Standard English pronunciation of 'feet' or 'tree'). In contrast, if the tongue lies flat and the lips are pursed, we produce an /u/ sound (as in Standard English 'spoon'). These different shapes alter how the vocal tract resonates and subtly change the pitch and qualities of the sound, enabling us to distinguish one vowel from another, independent of the speaker's own voice quality (e.g. Honda, 1983). You can hear this for yourself if you intone the sounds *oh, ooh, ah, eh, ee* on the same pitch: the fundamental frequency remains constant, but the vowel sounds become 'brighter' as the changing shape of the vocal tract causes specific frequencies to be emphasized. The shape and length of the vocal tract (from laryngeal height to lips) play a key role in the timbre of voice, even if the fundamental frequency is kept constant.

When the vocal system works to optimum conditions, voice quality is 'modal' (Laver, 1980). The vocal folds are in an ideal state of tension, and minimal breath pressure is needed for them to rapidly open and close. However, there are many interacting factors that can disrupt this process at the laryngeal level, and at levels above and below the larynx (Aronson & Bless, 2009; Sataloff, 2017). These include changes to aerodynamic functioning (breath control, breath pressure); differences in muscle tone and functional muscle control within the respiratory or vocal system; differences in the shape of the vocal tract and articulators; disorders of the vocal folds, such as stiffness, paralysis, inflammation, nodules or polyps, and neurological disorders that interfere with muscle movement. Any of these introduce imbalances, changing how the vocal folds oscillate and altering voice quality – a measure of how the voice sounds. For example, overly tense vocal folds can produce a harsh-sounding voice; vocal folds that remain open at one end can produce a breathy-sounding voice, and neurological disorders can lead to sudden changes in the muscles that control phonation, leading to a 'quavery' sounding voice. These types of difficulties in producing modal phonation are likely to affect children and young people who have muscle weakness, poor motor control or motor timing difficulties. Additionally, children and young people with anatomical differences are likely to have altered voice quality, as might those with some sensory differences. These factors are discussed in later sections in this chapter; but first, we will consider posture in relation to voice health.

THE INFLUENCE OF POSTURE ON VOICE

In the previous chapter, we discussed why posture can influence voice. In this section, we examine in more detail the way that poor posture within the head, neck and shoulders can affect voice production.

As described earlier in this chapter, the larynx is suspended within a network of muscles and ligaments. These enable it to move up and down when we swallow, move up for 'higher' vowel sounds, and descend for lower sounds. Because the larynx is connected to the hyoid bone, it is influenced by the position, movement and muscular tension of the jaw and tongue. From below, the muscles of the upper chest oppose the forces that lift the larynx. The position of the larynx and the way the voice is configured can be affected by atypical alignment of the upper body, especially, and by laxity or tension in any of these muscle groups. As physiotherapist Tracey Gjertsen explains, our neck and shoulder position is critical for voice production, but the position of our lower spine (the lumbar region, or lower back) can also affect our voice:

> The larynx is the primary organ of vocal function and its position in the anterior portion of the neck is directly dependent on the position of the head and shoulder girdle. A change in posture in the lumbar or thoracic spine will adversely affect the position of the neck and head and influence the mechanics of vocal production.

For ideal muscular balance and freedom, the vertebrae in the spine must be stacked neatly on top of each other, and the head should be balanced perfectly, its weight being distributed evenly across the neck and shoulders. Any alteration to the balance of muscles within the body has the potential to create long-term imbalances that affect and limit voice production (McCallion, 1998). A forward-head position, for example, brings the weight of the head forwards, and we must alter the whole of our posture to counter-balance this weight. This can lead to changes in the spine's shape, and – as we saw in Chapter 6 on breath – to changes in how the respiratory muscles function. Tracey Gjertsen explains why sitting or standing with a slumped posture is especially problematic:

> A common postural adaptation is a slumped thoracic spine which forces the head forwards of the shoulder line. As the cartilaginous structures of the larynx rely on soft tissue for their support, this type of postural deviation can disrupt voice production. It also disrupts

breathing. A forward head position causes expansion of the upper thoracic cage and compression in the lower thoracic region. This causes reduced respiratory function (Koseki *et al.*, 2019). In children, a forward head posture accompanied by mouth breathing reduces exercise capacity and lowers MIP and MEP (Okuro *et al.*, 2011).

As Tracey explains, a forward head changes the shape of the larynx and pharynx, altering resonance, and affects how easily we can control breath pressure for voice. If the habit is prolonged, the muscle that attaches the hyoid bone to the base of the skull can shorten, elevating the larynx, reducing its mobility and full access to the vocal range. Over time, poor postural habits limit voice production and can cause permanent damage.

SO WHAT CAN GO WRONG?

This section gives a brief overview of the main types and causes of voice disorders. The section highlights the range of possible factors that can affect voice and offers examples that may be more commonly found in people with sensory or developmental differences. However, some symptoms can arise from more than one cause: further reading is recommended (e.g. Aronson & Bless, 2009), and oversight from a professional is recommended if you are uncertain of the cause.

Main types of voice disorder

Voice disorders are usually categorized into functional, organic and neurological categories.

We will begin with *functional* voice disorders because these can arise from a young age in people with developmental and sensory differences. Functional voice disorders occur from inefficient phonation or misuse. The vocal structure is normal, but the child or young person might use too little muscular tension or excessive tension or force. Some functional voice disorders are psychological in origin; for example, emotions such as stress and anxiety can affect the voice, leading to excessive tension or weakness in phonation. Although there may be different causes for hyperfunction, the symptoms are similar: people tend to tighten their neck muscles, they may raise their larynx and may contract the muscles in their oesophagus, leading to the use of the false vocal folds. The voice may sound effortful and squeezed, strained, breathy or croaky. Over time, hyperfunction can cause organic problems. Any child or adult might develop functional voice disorders, but these have been commonly reported in children and adults with *ADHD* and *Down syndrome*. In Video 6 of the online resources you can see an example of ventricular phonation that is the likely result of excessive muscle tension.

Organic disorders occur when a physical or physiological condition affects the vocal folds, respiratory system or larynx. These include *structural differences* in the vocal folds, such as nodules, tumours or damage to the vocal folds. People who are susceptible to repeated respiratory infections may be at risk of damage to the vocal folds; for example, chronic inflammations or coughing can lead to damage; conditions such as gastrointestinal reflux (GERD) can cause laryngeal damage when the acid from the stomach repeatedly comes in contact with the vocal folds, and some medications – including asthma inhalers – or conditions such as POTS can dry out the vocal folds and tissues, which reduces the efficiency of the vocal folds and can cause speakers to use too much force (Fedorowski, 2018; Lechien *et al.*, 2019). Such conditions may occur in any child or young adult, but those with *cerebral palsy*, *Down syndrome*, *autism* and *ADHD* may be especially prone to respiratory infection; people with *cerebral palsy*, *Down syndrome* and *HSD/EDS* are also prone to GERD.

Neurological voice disorders arise from problems in the central nervous system. For example, the brain or the nerves may affect the function of the respiratory system, larynx or vocal folds and lead to disruption in the muscles needed for phonation, even though there might not be a problem within the muscles. Examples include spasmodic dysphonia, in which the muscles in the larynx suddenly contract (Aronson & Bless, 2009). Neurological causes are likely to affect people with *cerebral palsy* and may contribute to voice difficulties in people with *Down syndrome* and people who *stutter*.

Combinations and interactions

Any child, young person or adult can develop *functional* or *psychogenic voice disorders*. Some people might have voice disorders that fall into all categories – for example, misuse can lead to nodules and damage; or someone with a neurological voice disorder might overcompensate, leading to functional disorders. It can be challenging to identify specific causes of voice disorders in people with *cerebral palsy*, *Down syndrome* or *HSD/h-ESD*, as many factors affect different parts of the vocal system.

For example, these conditions can directly affect laryngeal function, but they also affect respiration and control of the breath pressure. In addition, differences within the oral cavity – such as poor muscle tone or muscle weakness, or anatomical differences (such as *cleft palate*) – can make it hard for someone to use their soft palate for voice and speech – this causes excess air to escape through the nose and affects the ability to control breath pressure for phonation. Some forms of therapy are successful for such complex voice disorders. For example, the Lee Silverman Voice Therapy training has been used to improve phonation in people with *cerebral palsy* (Pennington *et al.*, 2018). This improves motor control of voice by using increased volume during phonation, requiring the vocal and respiratory systems to work harder, and improving somatosensory and auditory feedback. However, careful oversight of such therapies is needed to avoid further damage and misuse.

Voice development and hormonal influences

The voice and vocal structure change as we age, with the most noticeable changes occurring at puberty and older age. As children age, the shape and positioning of the vocal tract change, and the muscles mature. When we are born, our larynx is high in the throat. Over the first year of life, the larynx begins to descend into the throat, altering the ratio between the volumes of the pharyngeal space and the vocal tract: this lowers the vocal pitch. The different components of the larynx continue to mature during childhood. The vocal folds also change: the vocal folds begin to develop layers between one and four years of age, and, gradually, the nerve fibres that help control the vocal folds start to increase in density. Partly because of these anatomical and physiological differences, younger children have a different vocal range from older children and adults, and do not have complete control over some aspects of their voice function (Welch, 2005).

Hormonal changes around puberty affect the structure and function of voice in boys and girls. For boys, hormonal changes cause an increase in the size of the larynx and lengthen the vocal folds. These changes cause their voice to drop by about an octave. Changes are less noticeable for female voices, but the menstrual cycle can impact their voice. Some women are especially sensitive to the effects of changing oestrogen levels, which can alter voice quality during their monthly cycle.

Although effects are subtle, hormonal changes can alter the neuro-muscular control of vocal folds and affect the timing for speech. Some may try to compensate for voice fluctuations, increasing their risk of developing functional voice disorders. For males with *Down syndrome*, for example, voice difficulties seem to be more prevalent after puberty than in childhood. The reason is unclear (Albertini *et al.*, 2010). Specific care may be needed to help those at risk of voice difficulties – such as children with *ADHD, autism, Down syndrome, cerebral palsy, HSD/h-EDS* – as they undergo these changes. For females, it may be necessary to monitor voice function across several months to identify any patterns. If in doubt, seek guidance from a health professional about how to protect the voice during these vulnerable times.

Emotions and voice

Voice and emotion are deeply connected in terms of evolution, function and communication. As infants, we are soothed or roused by the voices of our caregivers, friends and family and we soon learn that our voice inspires others to action. We communicate emotions such as hunger and distress through primal vocalizations; we can self-soothe by playing with the sound of our voice. As we grow, our vocal tone, volume and intonation can all help signal our meaning and emotional state. But our voice function is also affected by our emotional state, even if we are unaware of it (e.g. Johnstone & Scherer, 1999). People who are depressed or anxious tend to use less of their vocal range than someone feeling happy or excited. We can find our voices breaking when we are upset, anxious, angry or fearful, and powerful emotions can interfere with our ability to produce a voice at all. Stress and anxiety, especially, have significant effects on phonation. Because they produce physiological states that affect our whole body. For example, as we prepare for 'fight or flight', a stress response that developed to support us in life-or-death situation, we automatically brace our upper bodies for combat and increase our heart rate. A side-effect of this is that our voices tend to rise in pitch and become less 'smooth'; we may contract our external laryngeal muscles, causing our voices to become rough and harsh or disappear altogether. Our voices are so sensitive to emotions like stress that they change when we are under cognitive load – if we cause people to work under pressure by increasing the complexity of tasks they must perform, their voices show signs of stress. In my research, I found that people with *Down syndrome* showed very clearly the effects of stress and cognitive load in their voice (Jeffery, 2016). If I asked them to repeat words that exceeded their auditory memory, or reading tasks that required extra attention, their voices and speech would change: their voice quality would become more harsh or breathy; they might experience voice 'breaks', where the voice would stop briefly; or they might stutter. (See Video 6 in the online resources to see and hear an example of how cognitive load affected Andrew's voice.) When working with people who are already at risk of voice difficulties, especially those who find using words difficult, the sound of their voice or the absence of their voice may be a clear signal of their emotional state and an indication of stress.

HOW TO HELP YOUNG PEOPLE
DEVELOP A HEALTHY VOICE
General principles

It is important to understand the range of factors that can affect phonation in all children and young adults and the risks associated with a specific type of need. We will consider particular risks in the next chapter, but some general principles can be applied to support phonation for all voices:

- Aim to maintain good alignment of the head, neck and spine when using voice.
- Keep the voice hydrated.
- Monitor for tension in the shoulder and neck area.
- Be aware of sensitivity to changes in the environment: dust, pollen, pollutants, heating and medications.
- Be aware of sensitivity to changes in the body, especially hormonal influences.
- Be aware that cognitive and emotional stress can all trigger or exacerbate difficulties in phonation.

Establishing a breath-body-voice connection

The next step in breathwork and posture is to combine these elements with phonation. Chapter 8 will explore the nature of voice difficulties and give exercises to strengthen the voice. However, you can build on the above principles and the breathing activities in Chapter 6 to encourage the coordination between the breath and the voice. Once a child or young person is in a good posture for breathing and has learned to control their breath for non-vocal activities, you may begin to combine these skills. Begin with simple vocal exercises that allow them to connect the breath with the voice: observe for any changes in their posture (if they are seated or still) or changes in muscular tension, especially in the head-neck area. You might experiment with soft-onsets by adding a puff of breath at the start of a vowel – such as 'ha' or 'hoo' sounds. 'Yawn-sigh' exercises are also helpful in connecting breath and phonation. Adding /h/ or /y/ sounds to a humming sound can also help people find their voice without using too much effort – for example, you might discuss their favourite foods and encourage a 'yumm' sound. You can also experiment with 'hung' to encourage movement in the soft palate, as it seals the mouth cavity, allowing the sound to escape through the nose. Watch out for additional tension in the throat area during humming or 'ng' sounds – especially in anyone who has developed a habit of contracting their throat muscles to sing or speak. Humming exercises do help reduce muscle tension in children and adults, so if you notice ongoing tension, ask the child or young person to try the following:

1. Stretch and contract the face muscles, by opening the mouth and eyes (as in an expression of surprise) and sticking out the tongue; then retract the tongue and close and squeeze the face.
2. Gently massage the lower jaw, including under the jaw line.
3. Practise any of the above, and encourage them to feel the vibration in their mouth, lips or nose: you can ask them to put their hands over their face to feel it; you might also ask them to wear headphones to increase the auditory feedback they receive.
4. Use a rising humming movement – um-hum – at different pitches.

Once you can establish a soft-onset continuous sound, such as a humming noise, you can incorporate this into breath and posture work, or use it as a relaxation or sound awareness activity. Humming sounds are an important part of some yoga and meditation practices, and support feelings of relaxation and calm, meditative states and feelings of connection with others. It may be helpful to use such techniques as part of a warm-up or cool-down to music work, especially when working with groups. For example, in her book *Constructing Musical Healing*, June Boyce-Tillman (2000) describes several exercises that encourage both sound awareness and a meditative state using humming. In one example, each member of the group lies in a circle, with their heads forming the inner circle, like spokes on a wheel. You sound a gong to begin, and as its sound fades, direct them to hum at any note (remind them to breathe and refresh their hum!). After a while, ask them to change their humming note – can they, as a group, find a sound that works in harmony, or that sounds particularly pleasing? Tillman recommends using Indian cymbals as a cue for the voices to begin to quieten and fade; then finish with another gong, and all listen as its sound fades towards silence.

You can adapt this to create a sound bath, by placing a child or young person in the centre of a humming group, or by conducting the humming on a large resonant board. Ask them to close their eyes and listen to the sound – you could ask the learner to help you conduct the sound; for example, ask them to signal/gesture to you when it sounds good to them, or if they need it louder or quieter, or use your own observations of their expressions as cues. If you are working in a group with learners who are not yet verbal, this is a good way to involve them in the activity.

CHAPTER SUMMARY

As we have seen, the human voice is a complex construct: to work well, its constituent parts within the larynx and the body need to be in balance. Although the voice is robust, it is easy to upset the balance, and, over time, this can lead to damage. With awareness, we can control some of the factors that affect voice: for example, we can do all we can to strengthen and support the postural muscles and develop an awareness of unnecessary and unhelpful tension. We can also keep the voice well hydrated, which helps keep the mucosal linings of the voice and throat working smoothly. However, some causes of voice disorder are complex and may be less easy to address. Additionally, there can be considerable overlap between symptoms and causes. Our primary aim when working with young people on their voice is to instil good postural habits, avoid poor functional habits and maintain a healthy environment for the voice itself, physiologically and emotionally. Beyond this, specialist advice and input may be needed. There are also adaptations we can make to support voice function for specific physiological and sensory needs, and these will be discussed in the next chapter.

RECOMMENDED READING AND RESOURCES

Boyce-Tillman, J. (2000). *Constructing Musical Healing: The Wounds that Sing*. London: Jessica Kingsley Publishers.

Kayes, G. & Fisher, J. (2016). *This Is a Voice: 99 Exercises to Train, Project and Harness the Power of Your Voice*. London: Wellcome Collection.

The Voice Foundation – this website has information about voice science, voice disorders and health, including free videos and lectures: https://voicefoundation.org/health-science/videos-education/#VoiceDisorders.

Vocal Process – a website run by Gillyanne Kayes and Jeremy Fisher. These experienced voice coaches and doctors have many resources about the voice and how it works, and offer detailed training: https://vocalprocess.co.uk. They also have instructions to make a tilting larynx here: https://vocalprocess.co.uk/build-your-own-tilting-larynx.

CHAPTER 8

Understanding and Supporting Voice Difficulties

THE BIG QUESTIONS

What difficulties might someone I work with have when they use their voice? How can I help them overcome some of these difficulties using singing and music activities?

By the end of the chapter, you will:

- know how some physiological, sensory and cognitive differences can affect voice health and function in singing and speech
- know some general approaches to support voice function and health through singing
- know how to adapt commonly used vocal-strengthening activities to reduce the effects of some sensory or physiological needs.

WHO IS THIS FOR?

This chapter is relevant to people with sensory processing differences (such as those with auditory processing difficulties, autism, ADHD), hearing loss, and people with a combination of physiological and sensory differences such as *Down syndrome*, *cerebral palsy* or *hypermobile spectrum disorders/EDS*.

Chapter 7 introduced different types of voice disorders and identified how different groups could be at increased risk of voice difficulty. This chapter builds on this, offering further explanation and detail of common risks, and giving clear examples that show how complex these issues can be. We will focus on the physiological aspects of voice in people with *hypermobility spectrum disorders* and *Down syndrome*, then consider how sensory processing difficulties and hearing loss can affect voice. Once you understand the range of causal and exacerbating factors, you can address factors that are known to aggravate voice difficulties, if appropriate, or know when to seek specialist advice. The chapter concludes with examples of vocal activities and exercises easily incorporated into musical activities and known to support and strengthen phonation. There are also suggestions for how activities might be adapted to support postural control and minimize additional risk.

We will begin by comparing how we use our vocal structures when speaking or singing – this will help us understand some of the ways that singing can 'exercise' voice for speech and support voice function.

WHY MIGHT SINGING HELP THE SPEAKING VOICE?

In Chapter 7, we looked at the physiological processes needed for voice. We use the same physiological processes for singing but there are differences in how the vocal organs are set up or configured: we know this intuitively and set our voice in different ways to perform different tasks without giving it conscious thought. For example, if we intend to shout to someone in another room, before we make the first sound we might drop our jaw, raise the soft palate at the back of the mouth, widen the space above the larynx. The effect of this – relative to producing the same sound at conversational level – is to increase resonance, or the ability of the voice to 'carry', and volume. If, when calling, we sustain some sounds, we are effectively singing. But what singing adds to calling is precise tuning of notes and the ability to move rapidly between notes across an extended pitch range.

In conversational speech, we use a relatively limited pitch range, only using our wider pitch range when emphasizing a word or syllable, or when we are in a heightened emotional state. We use the least effort when speaking within the lower third of our range. In contrast, singing habitually draws on a much wider pitch range than we use for speaking. An untrained child or adolescent singer with a healthy voice can sing (pitch notes) across approximately 24 semitones (Dienerowitz *et al.*, 2021). This act requires several parts of the vocal apparatus to move beyond their habitual speaking state. Depending on the desired pitch and tone, the arytenoids (see Chapter 7, Figure 7.3) may open more widely and the larynx lift, lower or tilt to alter the length and thickness of the vocal folds. Almost simultaneously, with the vocal folds closed, the intercostal muscles will open the ribs (see Chapter 6) to generate a change in sub-glottal pressure that will produce voice at the desired volume without altering the vocal pitch; and this pressure will be controlled for the duration of the note to allow the singer to change volume or tone. These movements are learned through experience, from somatosensory feedback and from the responses of others. Control comes with practice and with maturation of the relevant muscles and organs.

One difference between speaking and singing, then, is physiological. It lies in the degree of activation of the muscles that are involved. (Another difference is psychological – we will examine this in Chapter 9.) In singing, parts of the vocal apparatus are working at greater degrees of stretch, relaxation or tension than when speaking. This is one reason that singing may act as a form of physical therapy for the speaking voice: singing may be more physically demanding on some of the small muscles involved, and this act may help them to increase strength, endurance and flexibility in the same way as any other physical workout. It is this 'over-training' in physiological processes and in rhythmic timing and pitching that can lead to changes in speech.

Singing can protect against loss of voice in some groups – for example, singing has helped people with neurological conditions such as Parkinson's to recover voice; it can support muscle weakness in voice and articulation in people with dysarthria; it can strengthen the voice and reduce risk of developing structural problems such as nodules; and it can reverse the effects of functional disorders (e.g. muscle tension dysphonia). The act of singing allows us to practise efficient vocal production and prolonged respiration. This has implications for the control of voice in producing voice contrasts in speech and for prosody. Rinta and Welch (2008) argue that singing may be particularly beneficial in the remediation of speech and voice disorders in pre-pubertal children.

However, the efficacy and suitability of singing activities for strengthening the voice depends on the nature of the voice difficulties and associated health conditions. We will now examine some of these complex issues and evaluate how – and if – singing can help.

VOICE DIFFERENCES AND DIFFICULTIES: UNDERSTANDING PHYSICAL DIFFERENCES AND COMPLICATIONS

We begin this section by looking at voice in people with hypermobile conditions. The information below focuses on people whose primary diagnosis is *hypermobility spectrum disorder* or *Ehlers Danlos syndrome*.

However, hypermobility disorders are commonly identified in children and young people with *autism*, *ADHD*, *dyspraxia*, *Down syndrome*, *fibromyalgia*, and some of the associated health conditions in people with *cerebral palsy*.

We will then look at voice function in people with *Down syndrome*, allowing us to consider how additional factors – such as working memory and cognitive load – can affect voice.

Hypermobility spectrum disorders and voice

People with hypermobile spectrum disorders have problems with their large muscles and joints, which typically result in joints that move beyond a normal range of movement. Over-stretchy or lax ligaments contribute to over-extension. These factors can result in joint instability, dislocations and subluxations in which the joint partially dislocates. However, the underlying cause of hypermobility is believed to be a connective tissue disorder, which affects the cellular structures of ligaments, tendons and tissues (Grahame, 1999). For this reason, hypermobility can affect the tissues, muscles and ligaments of the vocal system. An early survey showed that approximately 28 per cent of people with Ehlers Danlos syndrome have difficulties using their voice; this compared to approximately 28 in 100,000 of the general population who had dysphonia diagnoses (Hunter, Morgan & Bird, 1998). In 2020, I surveyed 273 adults with hypermobile conditions (HSD/h-EDS): 71 per cent reported having voice difficulties. In both surveys, people described sudden and intermittent loss of voice; hoarseness after speaking or singing; feelings of choking, pain, breathiness, strain; difficulties in controlling pitch, volume and breath; and becoming easily fatigued when talking or singing. Some people described problems in achieving volume and in controlling respiration. Despite having healthy lungs, and sometimes unusually large lungs, they seemed to run out of air too quickly.

The instability of joints in hypermobility is well documented, even in people who take great care to develop and strengthen muscle tone. The muscles and joints of the voice (see Chapter 7) are no exception. Several voice specialists have identified how the hypermobility of structures within the larynx can cause sudden difficulties, as they do in the large joints, such as knees, shoulders or hips. For example, the small cartilages that attach to the vocal folds (the arytenoids – see Figure 7.3 in Chapter 7) can sometimes partially dislocate and obstruct the airways (Arulanandam *et al.*, 2017; Safi *et al.*, 2017). Taking an in-breath can also be problematic, as the airways can be 'floppy', causing partial closure or obstruction of the airways. This gives symptoms that can be mistaken for asthma and treated as such with medication (Chatzoudis *et al.*, 2015). Some people with HSD/h-EDS find that the hyoid bone can also sublux, affecting the laryngeal structures that descend from it. Hypermobility in the upper neck can lead to excessive tipping back of the head, which can overstretch some vocal structures, and the vocal folds and small joints can over-extend similarly to other mobile joints and muscles.

We cannot alter ligamentous laxity that causes dislocations – we can only strengthen the muscles around a joint and teach awareness to help stabilize it. This is relatively easy in a large limb (e.g. a shoulder), whose movements can be seen and felt, but we might find it more challenging to feel and control the small muscles that support the voice. Theoretically, we might minimize the adverse effects of ligamentous laxity by strengthening the relevant muscles. For example, an exercise such as a simple 'siren' could support and strengthen the muscles needed to stabilize joints within the larynx.

In practice, singing can improve voice function, when combined with good technique. As one of my study participants (Jeffery *et al.*, 2021) explained, the voice can be developed when training works the body as well as the voice:

> My singing voice [...] transformed while at drama school, as my speaking voice transformed. Vocal techniques drawn on at drama school include those developed by Kristin Linklater, and Cis Berry, complemented by singing training for the actor. And fundamentally important; daily release work through the Alexander Technique, Tai Chi and Quigong, Laban, daily personalised vocal exercises that we were given to complete privately throughout our training. [...] My tutors worked meticulously with me [on my] voice, and sometimes progress was slower than expected – even basic things, like producing continuous sound for longer than 20 seconds, were initially problematic. But ultimately, they gave me my voice, and I use their teachings in my daily life. (Female singer with h-EDS)

Despite some positive outcomes like this, good singing technique was not always enough to alleviate ongoing vocal problems (Jeffery *et al.*, 2021). Many participants in my study attributed vocal symptoms to their medical conditions, such as *acid reflux*, *chronic fatigue*, *POTS/*

dysautonomia and *MAST cell disorders*. These commonly occur in connective tissue disorders and can prove challenging to manage. With acid reflux (or GERD), the acid that digests our food sometimes rises upwards into our larynx or pharynx. Over time, acid reflux can damage the vocal structures, causing inflammation and vocal nodules, limiting the vocal folds' ability to open and close efficiently. Likewise, dysautonomia can affect the voice directly, and indirectly. Dysautonomia is a disorder of the autonomic system; there are many sub-types, of which POTS is one. Dysautonomia can cause dehydration and reduced blood circulation, which can potentially affect the vocal folds and lead to voice problems. Dysautonomia, especially POTS, can also cause dizziness, fainting and feelings of anxiety or panic, especially when standing upright. As such, POTS can affect posture and breathing abilities when singing. Likewise, many of my participants described how MAST cell disorders triggered symptoms similar to asthma, affecting their airways and breathing abilities and potentially their voice. Even if these conditions do not directly affect the voice, they make it much harder for those with hypermobility to know *why* they cannot use their voice as well as they desire. These issues are unpredictable and cause many difficulties for singers, not least because they find it hard to obtain a diagnosis.

Little is currently understood about voice development in people with hypermobile conditions, or how to best support them. For you, as practitioners, parents or carers, the first step is simply to be aware of the risks:

- There may be hidden musculoskeletal or physiological complications that affect the vocal tract directly, the jaw or the breathing system. These can be intermittent and may cause pain.
- Acid reflux (GERD) can occur unnoticed (e.g. while sleeping), causing ongoing and untreated damage.
- The voice tires easily; over the long term, this can damage the vocal folds.
- MAST cell disorders and sensitivities to allergens might affect the vocal folds and respiratory tract.
- POTS can lead to problems using the voice, especially in upright positions, whether seated or standing.
- The vocal structures can be over-stretched, leading to increased risk of damage.
- The vocal organs may be slow to heal, once damaged.

In hypermobile children and young adults who show signs of voice prob-lems, it is essential to support the factors that can be easily controlled and managed – such as maintaining hydration, avoiding over-use of breathing muscles or over-extending the vocal range, and considering whether a seated or supine position might alleviate some symptoms. However, there can be physiological and medical factors to consider, too, so seek medical advice as necessary.

DOWN SYNDROME AND VOICE

Case study: Jack

Jack, aged 22 years, loves to sing everything from Disney to rock. He likes to talk, too, and finds speaking and reading aloud quite easy. He has a well-developed vocabulary and articulates most words with clarity. However, he finds it very hard to use his voice. He has difficulty making his voice start: he seems to squeeze it until it forces its way out, overly loud and forceful. It sounds as though it takes a lot of concentration and physical effort for him to speak. Sometimes, his singing voice also sounds harsh and stays very low in pitch; he cannot control pitch or melody, or sustain notes. Then it will suddenly break into a lighter voice, soft and falsetto. Suddenly, he has control over pitch and duration and can show his singing and musical abilities.

People with Down syndrome have distinctive voices. Listeners com-monly describe their voices as harsh, hoarse, gruff, breathy, low-pitched, high-pitched, nasal or a combination of these (e.g. see reviews by Kent & Vorperian, 2013; Krishnamurthy & Ramani, 2020). Some of these qualities are due to physiological differences that affect resonance. The smaller oral cavity and relatively large tongue of people with Down syndrome create a vocal tract that is subtly different in its shape from people without Down syndrome (see Figure 8.1). In addition, people with Down syndrome have low muscle tone. This affects the tissues within the oral cavity and pharyngeal walls, whose softness affects how the sound is reflected, dampening it. These anatomical and physiological characteristics contribute to the distinctive Down syndrome voice type. They also have difficulties moving the articulators (lips, tongue) and may find it difficult to move their soft palate or use their velopharyngeal muscles to isolate the nasal cavity from the mouth, which can create a more 'nasal' sounding voice (Beck, 2010). It is unclear how much of their voice quality or difficulty stems from problems controlling the vocal folds, as other physiological factors can affect phonation. For example, a loss of air through the nose can affect phonation as it changes the balance between supra- and sub-glottal pressure. Their voice can be affected by excessive nasal emission, restricted tongue movement, respiratory system differences, postural differences, such as a forward-head position, and mouth breathing, which can be caused by chronic upper respiratory infections and which dries out the mouth and larynx.

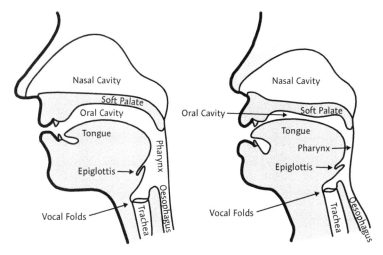

Figure 8.1: Anatomy of the vocal tract in a child with Down syndrome. The figure shows how the oral and vocal tract in a young person without Down syndrome (left) compares to that of someone with Down syndrome (right). The image is based on MRI scans of a young child and adult with Down syndrome (Rodrigues *et al.*, 2019). It shows how the oral cavity is smaller, making the tongue appear larger and placing it in a forward position within the mouth. The soft palate and uvula are slightly thicker and shorter, the nasal cavity is smaller and the trachea is narrower. These differences in shape can affect how the voice works, because of differences in air pressure at the glottis, and they change the resonance of the voice.

In addition to medical complications, people with Down syndrome have hypermobility and poor muscle tone. These can affect their external and intrinsic laryngeal muscles, including the vocal muscles. Pryce (1994), in studying the activation of the vocal cords in people with Down syndrome, concluded that reduced muscle tone causes people with Down syndrome to use more energy to activate their vocal cords.

The extra effort they need when producing voice may cause them to use more tension in their muscles, leading to *muscle tension dysphonia*. This can sometimes involve the oscillation of the false vocal folds (see Chapter 7) and higher structures within the larynx at the same time as the vocal folds, or instead of the vocal folds, resulting in a sound that is described in singing as 'growl'. Jack (above), Andrew (Chapter 4) and other adults with Down syndrome sometimes use this 'ventricular' phonation. This is likely to be a subconscious habit they developed to get the vocal folds moving due to their hypermobility and weaker vocal muscles. You can hear an example of ventricular phonation in Video 6 of the online resources.

Postural differences may also lead to altered tension within the vocal tract and compensatory muscle use, and this can all be complicated by other comorbid health conditions, including increased risk of heart disease, thyroid imbalance, GERD and recurring respiratory infections (Mitchell, Call & Kerry, 2003; Ramia *et al.*, 2014). Physiotherapist Tracey Gjertson explains some of these complexities:

> Respiratory muscle weakness is common in conditions where hyper-mobility or low muscle tone occur. Poor cardiorespiratory fitness affects participation in activities of daily living and is likely to cause secondary health conditions such as recurrent chest infections, pneumonia and stroke. People with Down syndrome demonstrate a 50 per cent reduction in MEP and MIP, coupled with poor postural tone and endurance; in fact, respiratory tract infections cause 40 per cent of the hospital admissions for children with Down syndrome (Keles *et al.*, 2018). It is important to note that obstructive airway anomalies are common in Down syndrome and although speech and singing programmes may improve voice and respiratory function, they may be too effortful for some.

Differences in the larynx and pharynx contribute to a distinctive voice quality, but people with Down syndrome can have more difficulty producing modal phonation when under pressure to perform a task. Their voice can break down when they imitate words or phrases that exceed their memory span, which is often very short (e.g. see Chapter 2). If we teach by imitation – for example, when teaching the words to a song – we must consider how to reduce the length and complexity of words or phrases. Keeping voice tasks as simple as possible will reduce the amount of information someone with Down syndrome must process, and this will improve conditions for phonation. We will return to these principles in Chapter 9.

Finally, the same types of developmental and hormonal changes that affect phonation in typically developing children (see Chapter 6) will affect children and young people with Down syndrome. People with Down syndrome seem to have more difficulty using their voices after puberty (Albertini *et al.*, 2010). Therefore, additional care may be needed during the transition to adolescence to set up habits in relaxed posture and identify and reduce any habits that introduce tension in the throat, jaw, shoulders or breathing muscles.

SENSORY DIFFERENCES AND VOICE

When we use our voice to speak or sing, we draw on multisensory feedback from our ears and body. As the vibrating air resonates within the oral cavities and larynx, our brain receives subtle signals about how the voice feels and how it sounds. This feedback allows us to monitor and adjust our voice – this happens incredibly quickly and without overt, conscious control. If we direct conscious attention to these feelings and sounds, we can manipulate the voice further. We can deliberately add 'bright', 'twangy' or 'deeper' overtones through conscious monitoring and 'placement' of the voice. This process of receiving and interpreting multisensory feedback can be reduced or altered in people with sensory loss or sensory processing differences that affect auditory and physiological perception.

The perception of voice will be altered in people with *auditory processing differences*. As we explored in Chapter 1, a child, young person or adult with sensory differences might have very different sound experiences to us. This can affect how they hear their own voice and external sounds. For people with auditory processing difficulties, the feedback from their own voice via their ears may be distorted, unclear or delayed, or appear overly loud. Altered auditory feedback can have significant consequences for phonation and voice control. For example, people with hearing loss can have difficulty controlling loudness and pitch. Likewise, people change their voice function in response to auditory processing changes. If you change the auditory signal that reaches the ears of a singer as they sing a steady note – for example, by increasing or lowering the pitch – then the singer alters their own pitch to compensate.

For some people who have auditory processing differences, the altered perception of their own voice can lead to symptoms of dysphonia, such as a hoarse, weak or breathy sounding voice, or a tendency to strain or use too much force to activate the voice.

For people with difficulties processing internal physical feelings (*interoception*), the biofeedback from vibrations and subtle laryngeal movements may be missing, altered or delayed. Most of us can feel and control the relatively large movements we use for speaking and breathing – such as the movements of our lips, tongue, soft palate and ribs. However, altered feedback from these muscles can affect voice production and voice quality. If the signal from these muscles is weak, our movements may become less precise, or we might use too much tension in the muscle. The small motor movements that control phonation rely partly on the development of automatic planning at a neurological level and muscle memory. Recent studies with people who have *muscle tension dysphonia* have shown unusual activation in brain areas associated with muscle control and altered feedback during phonation (e.g. Kryshtopava *et al.*, 2017). It is, therefore, possible that altered sensory perception can lead to abnormal muscle tension and disturbances to phonation.

People with *hearing loss* will experience their voice differently from people with full hearing, and will have different methods of controlling their voice. Hearing loss affects the auditory feedback loop that occurs via the ears – some parts of the voice signal will be missing, or low in volume or quality. Depending on the type and extent of hearing loss, a speaker may rely more on feedback from the bones in the head than on sound transmitted in the air – the bones also resonate as voice is produced and can be 'heard' through bone conduction. Partly because of the altered feedback process, people with hearing loss are at risk of voice production difficulties. Without as much feedback from hearing, they might use high levels of sub-glottal pressure to kick-start their voice. This can increase the somatosensory feedback during phonation, but it can result in a higher-pitched voice and, over time, damage the vocal folds (Hocevar-Boltezar, 2006). They might also have noticeable 'breathiness' and have problems with breath control for voice. However, children with cochlear implants may have better vocal control, as the implants help them monitor the sound quality more easily (Mathur & Banik, 2015). This reduces the risks of long-term damage. (NOTE: Jack, above, also had an unconfirmed level of hearing loss; this will be another factor that influenced his voice quality and volume.)

Case study: Mira

Mira sings all the time. She is a natural mimic, with a clear sense of fun and an aura of confidence. She often initiates communication with others by singing songs and extracts of dialogue from movies. Sometimes she re-enacts elements, too: she might greet someone with an imaginary sword thrust and a holler, drawn straight from her favourite film.

Mira is an exuberant singer. Her voice is loud, resonant, well tuned and within key. He is quick to pick up words, melody and rhythm; she can reproduce a new song with just one or two repetitions, and she accepts variations to words and key if these are introduced in the first few listens. Mira is beginning to learn how to control her volume and tone for singing. Some of her peers, who also have autism, sing with a subtlety that brings audiences to tears; but for Mira, who evidently feels and responds to the emotion of songs, conveying this through her voice is a skill that she is yet to develop.

Many people with autism use their voices for singing even if they do not speak. Some are excellent mimics but can struggle with changes to key, tune or words, and some are creative vocalists who bring their own character to a favourite song. Others are enthusiastic in their singing, but have difficulties in controlling some aspects of their voice, like Mira. She has developed some vocal habits that can damage her voice over time, and that restrict her range when singing. To help her improve, we need to understand more about how she learns and how we can teach her.

Some children, adolescents and adults with autism speak or sing with distinctive voice quality (e.g. Fusaroli, 2021; Shriberg *et al.*, 2001). Researchers have struggled to explain why. Some have reported subtle acoustic differences in how newborn infants with autism use their voices, suggesting that their voice qualities might be present from birth (Sheinkopf *et al.*, 2012; Unwin *et al.*, 2017). Older children can have voices that sound overly nasal, overly loud or forceful, or atypical in pitch (Patel *et al.*, 2019). Some vocal differences might stem from differences in how young children with autism develop joint attention or an understanding of emotional cues (Sheinkopf *et al.*, 2012). Other research indicates that they might not find voices as interesting as infants without autism (Sperdin & Schaer, 2016), which will make all vocal learning more challenging. For example, brain studies show that infants with autism receive lower signals of pleasure or reward when listening to voices (Blasi *et al.*, 2015). These explanations remind us that some learners will get no pleasure from singing or using their voice, or listening to ours. We should be aware of this possibility – especially if the young person is one of a large group – and offer them non-vocal ways to take part (e.g. by using instruments, props, movements, or just sitting this one out).

There is still much to understand about sound perception in people with autism, especially given that auditory sensitivity varies between individuals. However, auditory processing differences are commonly reported in children and adults with autism, along with other types of sensory processing differences. Altered auditory processing can affect voice perception and voice production. Whereas most typically developing people can hear if a singer wavers in pitch by just a 2 per cent change in fundamental frequency, people with autism are less sensitive to pitch changes in voice (O'Connor, 2012). However, they can usually detect small changes in pitch in non-vocal sounds. Experiments with children with autism have shown that when auditory feedback is disrupted their voices will become either more monotone or more variable in pitch (Patel *et al.*, 2019). So altered feedback may explain why some children and young people with autism use pitch differently when speaking.

Furthermore, some people with autism might process the somatosensory signals from their voice differently from their neurotypical peers. As we saw in Chapter 3, sensory differences and differences in integrating streams of sensory information can affect movements. In the same way that sensory integration difficulties affect timing for drumming (e.g. Chloe, Chapter 2), it will be hard for someone to control their phonation and pitch if the signals from their body and ears are not smoothly processed or integrated. In practical terms, children and young people with autism and other processing difficulties might find it difficult to sustain controlled phonation. This will be even more difficult against a background of other sound, such as another person singing, or music.

People with *ADHD* may also experience problems caused by atypical auditory processing and altered somatosensory processing. Some research suggests that children with ADHD might be more susceptible to vocal hyperfunction than their peers (Barona-Lleo & Fernandez, 2016). Specifically, they might use too much muscular energy to produce their voice. As a result, they are at greater risk of developing vocal nodules.

However, not all researchers agree that ADHD is a risk factor for voice difficulties. To date, no research has untangled the various effects that these separate issues may have for voice production in children with ADHD. For practice, it is worth assuming that any of these challenges associated with ADHD could affect voice, and to take steps to reduce their effects; for example, by watching for excessive laryngeal tension, supporting the person's awareness of their voice, and by giving and enabling feedback in multisensory formats, rather than relying on auditory feedback only.

Supporting the voice of people with sensory processing differences will need a tailored approach, based on their needs and preferences. It might be helpful to use non-verbal feedback to help a child to control their voice. For example, you might use a visual signal to indicate loudness rather than expecting them to rely on auditory feedback alone. It is also important to consider the wide range of factors that could affect voice production and quality in a child or young adult with autism. Let us consider a child who has autism + hypermobility + auditory processing difficulties. This child may have some difficulty in processing vocal pitch or quality. Additionally, the signal that reaches their ears may be delayed. This can interrupt and interfere with their voice production, affecting their pitch and tone control. Their hypermobility might affect their vocal system; this, too, may affect regulation of pitch and tone, as well as breath control, and could increase the risk of using excessive muscle tension when talking or singing. Furthermore, the child may receive anxiety-like or anxiety-producing signals from their body because of a heightened nervous system. Singing at volume may be one way for this child to soothe their nervous system – as singing promotes longer exhalations, thereby calming the fight-or-flight response, and as physical sensations that come from singing loudly may help mask other incoming sensory signals.

The way we support the hypothetical child above would be very different from how we support another child who has autism but lacks hypermobility, or one who has hyposensitivity to auditory information and hypersensitivity to touch. Given the scarcity of research that focuses on developing voice and phonation in people with complex and comorbid differences, cautious experimentation may be key, with the support of speech and language therapists.

HOW CAN WE SUPPORT VOICE FUNCTION THROUGH SINGING?

Some voice disorders cannot be improved or removed by singing; indeed, singing might worsen organic disorders, such as nodules. If a child or young person has organic or neuromuscular vocal disorders (see Chapter 7), the aim would be to ensure that no damage is done when singing. Similarly, it is unclear how effective voice exercises can be for strengthening or healing the voice of a child or young person who has multiple medical issues. For children and young people at risk of hypermobility (such as those with Down syndrome, autism, ADHD) or at increased risk of acid reflux (such as those with cerebral palsy, Down syndrome), even careful voice training and care might not offset the risks posed by joint instabilities, over-stretching of vocal ligaments, or damage from acid reflux – or from the medications used to treat associated conditions, such as asthma. Unless you have specific guidance from a voice professional, avoid over-extending vocal range, maintain good hydration to reduce the effects of medication or acid, and continue to support postural stability.

The following general principles apply to all voices that are at increased risk of functional or emotional voice difficulties. These should be used with the principles outlined in Chapters 6 and 7:

- Gently 'stretch' the voice range but be aware of any changes in physical tension or posture when approaching high or low notes: if in doubt, keep within a medium range.
- Gently exercise the neck, shoulders, lower jaw and articulators, especially the tongue, which is connected – via the hyoid – to the larynx. Tension in the tongue root can inhibit laryngeal movement, lead to undesired tension in the voice, and inhibit vocal range. However, take care with jaw movements in hypermobile groups, as they can often experience jaw pain and full or partial dislocations. Gentle massage can help release muscle tension in these areas (Goffi-Fynn & Carroll, 2013).
- Aim to incorporate postural awareness into vocal exercises, but also consider using mobility aids, or other adaptations as advised by a physiotherapist, to stabilize vulnerable muscle groups. Asking young people to monitor posture and breathing and voice may create excessive cognitive load.

- Keep notes/a diary to identify any patterns in phonation – for example, in relation to stress, anxiety, tiredness, hormonal changes, medication.
- Explore voice function from different postural positions to eliminate the effects of tension, POTS or anxiety associated with 'performing'.
- Look for ways to reduce cognitive load so that attention can be directed to phonation: you might consider using cards and pictures as prompts for sounds; reduce sensory feedback from the environment.
- Consider the use of headphones during phonation – these will alter the sound of the voice, placing emphasis on vibrations from bone conduction; they may also help cut out extraneous noise; people may be able to use a louder voice with headphones on without 'forcing' the voice.
- Incorporate visual feedback of voice – apps and computer programs can give visual feedback about the quality of phonation, and can show changes in pitch and in quality (e.g. spectrum). Some are free (e.g. *Praat*). Visual feedback can be used to show when 'good' phonation is produced; it allows the person to experiment with small changes (e.g. posture) and see the difference this makes.
- Use somatosensory or tactile feedback (touch, vibration) to support perception of volume and pitch. Resonance boards and resonant props (balloons) or instruments (guitars, drums) can all be used to feel and hear vibrations produced by the voice at different volumes.
- Use microphones and amplification – these can improve confidence and reduce the drive to 'force' the voice. The amplification of the voice can support learners with hearing impairments and improve phonatory control.
- Experiment with approaches and combinations to learn what works best: for some, a microphone and amplification may work best while the singer wears headphones that are *not* connected to the amplified sound. Headphones can be used this way to mask external noise, increase feedback of the voice via bone conduction and to help socially anxious singers focus more on the feeling of singing than on the sound of their own voice.

In addition to supporting the voice, when used with care, singing offers multiple benefits to the body, and the emotions, too – it can help strengthen the muscles of respiration, the muscles that stabilize the core, can improve breathing and lung health, and flood the body with feel-good chemicals. The long out-breath used for singing can help calm the nervous system in a way that is similar to meditation. The children or young adults you work with do not need to be 'good' singers to benefit, or to even sing songs. Indeed, you can support voice production more easily if songs without words are used: this reduces cognitive load and helps you direct their focus to the element that you wish to improve, such as pitching, or reducing breathiness, volume, and so on.

Example vocal exercises and adaptations

Below are some vocal exercises based on those that have been successfully used in music therapy and voice therapy. The main aims of the activities are to address the types of problems common in people with sensory and physiological differences. The activities aim to improve vocal fold efficiency, improve soft onset of phonation (see also Chapter 7 – *Establishing a breath-body-voice connection*), reduce excessive tension when using voice, and provide feedback in multisensory ways. I include additional guidance about how to adapt them, and what to watch out for in children and adults with some of the complex sensory and physiological needs we have discussed. You can find more of these types of activities in the 'Recommended reading' section.

Table 8.1: Example vocal exercises and adaptations

Exercise	Exercise aim/function	Things to do more of	Things to reduce	Especially important for...
Using resonance tubes for vowels, sirens and nonsense words (semi-occluded vocal tract exercises)	Using resonance tubes (e.g. glass tubes, latex tubes, straws) changes the function of the larynx and makes it easier to produce efficient phonation without tension. Variations have been used to treat different voice disorders, depending on the diameter and length of the tube and the type of voice exercise. For more, see Simberg and Laine (2007) in 'Recommended reading' ('smart' and game versions are also being developed)	Aim for a good posture when doing this, and inhalation that expands the lower ribs	Lifting of shoulders, tightening of throat, short, tense in-breaths that lift shoulders	People at risk of developing voice disorders; breathy voices; voices that seem overly tense or harsh; people who need multisensory feedback – the bubbles provide visual cues about breath and voice, and the method can increase sensation in the throat. SOVT (semi-occluded vocal tract) techniques have also been successful in people with neurological voice disorders
/ng/ sounds and /m/ sounds	These allow for gentle phonation and produce different sensations; they exercise the soft palate		Watch out for 'squeezing' the voice – if in doubt, add an 'h' sound to encourage gentler onset	Checking and feeling velo-pharyngeal closure; supporting awareness of the soft palate
v/f + s/z exercises	Begin to connect the voice to breath; feel the connection as the epigastrium moves (see Chapter 6)	Encourage awareness of the physical movement as the breath moves; feel the difference at the larynx (e.g. fingers on larynx) between the voiced and voiceless sounds	Check that posture is maintained when vocalizing, and that the body does not slump out	Activating the voice without excessive tension and mobilizing the breathing

cont.

Exercise	Exercise aim/function	Things to do more of	Things to reduce	Especially important for...
Kazoo – 'sing' along to songs	Encourage soft phonation: using the kazoo needs the voice to work, and can promote an efficient voice sound	Check posture when singing but encourage movement	Check for signs of squeezing of the voice – you might encourage the learner to use their hands (to feel their neck) or a mirror to monitor for this	Kazooing along to favourite songs. This reduces the need to recall words and reduces cognitive load that can affect voice production
Singing into/ at a balloon or resonant instrument	Encourage volume and resonance – the vibrations can be felt (balloon, drum skin) or heard (stringed instrument)	Move the balloon/ resonator further away gradually and encourage 'bouncing' or 'throwing' the voice to it to reduce effort	Watch for tension or a change towards 'shouting' as volume increases	Providing tactile feedback about voice; it can augment auditory feedback
Lie on a wooden floor (or a resonance board) for vocal glides	Lying with arms spread wide, feel the vibration from the floor or board; focus on different body parts to feel the vibrations there	Experiment with different vowel sounds: some vowel sounds might be easier to produce or feel	Watch for hyperextension of body parts – support vulnerable areas, such as the knees, lower back or head, with cushions or rolled towels	Providing tactile feedback and reducing the strain of standing/ maintaining posture. The use of a resonance board may amplify sensations and increase somatosensory awareness
Imagine singing into different parts of the body and feel the resonance there	Feel or imagine the voice throughout the body	If appropriate, encourage the singer to use their hands to feel vibrations in parts of their body (e.g. head, throat, chest)		Imagining the sound in different parts of the body, which can change how the voice is produced; some might like the tactile feedback from feeling their voice resonate in their head bones or their sternum

Vocal sirens on vowels	A siren involves making a vocal sound between upper and lower vocal ranges – making these requires rapid changes in the length and thickness of the vocal folds, as they simultaneously open and close. This involves several sets of muscles and structures: the muscles controlling the arytenoid cartilages allow the vocal processes to pivot, thereby opening and closing the vocal folds at the back wall of the larynx; the thyroid cartilage at the front of the neck hinges forwards to stretch the vocal folds, causing them to tighten and raising the pitch. These movements are typically anchored by muscles that support and stabilize the larynx from the neck, upper chest, upper back and jaw	Aim to keep an even tone and volume, but listen for changes in parts of the range	Watch for tension in the throat or shoulders as pitch rises; watch for abdominal collapse in the lower pitch range or towards the end of the exercise	Caution is needed for those with hypermobility in laryngeal structures or with vocal folds that have been damaged to keep within safe parameters. For example, if a child is at risk of subluxations, or of irritating the vocal folds, keep within a range that does not over-extend the muscles and ligaments involved
Resonance boards	Sing while lying on a resonance board			People who struggle with maintaining an upright posture (e.g. due to POTS); depending on the sensitivity of the board and the resonance the singer produces, it can also provide somatosensory feedback. It can also be used by the practitioner to sing to the person on the board
Sing using cartoon voices	Using different voices, put the vocal mechanism into different configurations – this can help access new sounds and feelings and exercise the whole vocal tract			

CHAPTER SUMMARY

This chapter has identified why some children and young people can have difficulties in using their voice. It has considered how multiple health issues can contribute to voice difficulties in people with hypermobility spectrum disorders, how resonance and cognitive load can affect voice quality in people with Down syndrome, and how sensory processing issues can affect people with autism or ADHD. This chapter has also examined the potential of singing to support healthy voice production. It is not guaranteed that singing will reduce or reverse voice problems, especially if difficulties are organic. However, you may be able to prevent or reduce misuse if you can help children and young people develop good vocal (and postural) habits. Others with less complex conditions may benefit quickly from even simple exercises and attention to posture when singing. Developing good vocal habits for singing will help them free up more of their voice and support their voice for speaking.

RECOMMENDED READING

Corke, M. (2014). *Approaches to Communication through Music*. London: Routledge.

Simberg, S. & Laine, A. (2007). The resonance tube method in voice therapy: Description and practical implementations. *Logopedics Phoniatrics Vocology*, 32(4), 165–170.

CHAPTER 9

Using Singing and Songs for Speech

THE BIG QUESTIONS

How can singing and songs support early verbal skills? What types of difficulties might children and young people have with singing songs, and how can I develop their singing abilities? Can singing skills transfer to speech?

WHO IS THIS FOR?

You can use the ideas in this chapter with any child learning to sing and speak. However, the information is most relevant to children and adults who have difficulties producing speech sounds and words. You might use the ideas with people who have expressive challenges, such as *dyspraxia*, *dysarthria*, *stuttering/fluency* disorders or *cerebral palsy*. You can also use these ideas to learners with perceptual differences, including those with *hearing loss*, *auditory-memory difficulties* and *autism*.

By the end of this chapter, you will know:

- how most children learn to sing and how this relates to verbal learning
- why singing and songs can help your learner develop speech perception and production
- what you can do to help them sing new songs more easily
- where to look for more help in developing singing proficiency
- what an example of spontaneous transfer from song to speech looks like.

Chapter 8 examined how singing can support voice production; in this chapter, we consider why singing songs might be the most valuable form of verbal communication you can use to support speech and vocal communication. I begin by examining how most children learn to sing and how we differentiate speech from song. Although some acoustic cues help us tell apart song from speech, there is also ambiguity. I argue that some people with learning differences might not perceive speech and song as separate acts; as a result, they might find songs and song-like speech more appealing and motivating than adult-directed speech. We then focus on speech intelligibility. I discuss which aspects of speech and voice help us understand what another is saying and why and how singing can develop the skills that contribute to intelligibility. Next, I discuss the challenges that children and young people can face when singing songs or speaking, and I suggest how you can adapt activities so that learners can sing and learn songs more efficiently. I give examples of using songs and singing exercises to support specific aspects of speech.

HOW DO WE LEARN TO SING?

As we saw in Chapter 1, our connection with singing began in the womb. In the womb, the sound that reached our ears from any voice was all music: without the detail of consonants, we experienced a stripped-back form of language and song – just the melodic, rhythmic patterns of voice against the beat of our mother's heart. Nevertheless, this was a rich experience: it set us on our journey toward learning language and music (Chapter 3) and connected us emotionally with vocal sound and music (Welch, 2005).

In music and language, perception skills always develop before skills in production. Sometimes, there is a long gap between perceiving something and being able to reproduce it, especially when our cognitive and motor systems are immature. However, the baby begins to 'sing' from about two months of age. Newborns make a limited range of sounds because their vocal tract is shorter and their musculature is undeveloped. From about two to four months, the baby's motor systems and muscles mature, gaining more control over their voice. They exercise these muscles as they play with pitch, producing vocal sirens and glides. This stage of vocal learning is crucial in helping them master the prosody of their spoken language. They 'babble' at this stage, too. As they repeat streams of musical-sounding consonant-vowel patterns, they are working the articulatory, vocal and phonemic programmes they need for speech and song. From about four to seven months, this prosodic vocal play takes on characteristics of our mother language (see Welch, 2005 in 'Recommended reading and resources').

Infant-directed songs and speech play a role in developing a concept of tonality (e.g. the major and minor scales used in most Western music). When we speak or sing to babies, we produce relatively large melodic intervals common to musical cultures: thirds, fourths, fifths and octaves. Babies find these giant vocal leaps appealing, and they recognize that the patterns are meaningful because they hear them so much. Babies create tonal melodic patterns from about 19 months, beginning with small musical intervals of major seconds and minor thirds. By the age of two years, infants compose their own songs based on fragments of songs they already know and show evidence of a stable tonal centre (or 'key'). At this age, and until about four years, the child might use a singing-based form of communication, especially during play; young children do not necessarily separate speech and song. Towards school age, the child develops accuracy in rhythm and pitch as their motor and cognitive systems mature. At this age, too, they associate emotional states with major or minor tonalities and can create their own 'happy' and 'sad' songs.

Singing proficiency develops significantly between five and eleven years. However, no two children will develop accuracy in singing songs at quite the same rate; instead, they learn in phases, and some children may remain in one phase for longer than another. Researchers have developed two models to explain children's stages when learning to sing. Both models were based on extensive studies of children (Rutkowski, 1997; Welch, 1998). The studies showed that most children progress from 'speech-like chanting' of the text, through singing with a limited pitch range, to singing with a more comprehensive pitch range (Welch, 2016). These studies also showed that accurate singing depends on several complex factors, including age, sex and the nature of the task. Welch and colleagues discovered that children between five and eight years were more accurate singers if teachers broke a song into smaller tasks. They might focus on perfecting one element at a time, such as matching pitch or interval, or they might concentrate on the rhythmic pattern of phrases by replacing words with simple syllables (such as 'loo'). This deconstructed form helped boys and girls focus on the accuracy of pitch. However, the boys became less accurate than girls when reconstructing the song. As they aged, the singing skills of most boys in the studies remained behind those of the girls (Welch, 2016).

By the age of 11 years, 96 per cent of children can sing accurately. A large study by Welch *et al.* (2008) examined the singing proficiency of pupils aged between seven and ten years. The ten-year-olds were significantly more skilled than the seven-year-olds, confirming that singing ability develops with age. However, many social, cultural and experiential factors affect a child's singing development. These include their teacher's expectations, the learning environment, and how much the school values singing (Welch, 2009). During later childhood and adolescence, singing development is affected by the individual's view of singing and how they view themselves as a singer. At this age, especially, the type of feedback they receive from others is crucial; supportive and accurate feedback can increase the enjoyment of singing and improve their self-concept as a singer.

As we reach adulthood, our singing abilities depend on the number of hours we practise and how well we maintain our skills. After all, our voice depends on the strength, tone and agility of many muscles (see Chapter 7), which can atrophy without practice. Even if our voice remains in good shape, our performance can suffer if we place too many demands on our processing abilities and memory. For example, lengthy lyrical texts, dynamic changes and physical movements can cause us to lose our accuracy in pitch and timing. All of us can learn songs more easily if tasks are broken down and we take steps to reduce cognitive load while learning (Han, 2021). As adults, we master songs in incremental stages, which reduces the cognitive load. Typically, we first reproduce the approximate melodic and rhythmic 'shape' of the piece, then, we learn the words, next we gradually master the finer details of rhythm and pitch. We might need to make this process more overt or break the task into smaller steps for some songs or some learners.

HOW CAN SINGING SUPPORT VERBAL LEARNING?
The speech-song spectrum: can singing support verbal learning more efficiently than talking?

In Chapter 8, we considered how physiological and acoustic features help us to distinguish singing from conversational speech. The cues that make us perceive a sound as more 'song-like' than 'speech-like' include sustained pitches, elongated vowels, precise rhythmic patterning, discrete pitches and tonality. However, the distinction between speech and song is more in our minds than in the signal's acoustic features. Under certain conditions, we perceive *speech* as a song. The music psychologist, Dr Diana Deutsch, first described this 'speech-to-song' illusion (Deutsch, 2003). She discovered that for non-musicians, as few as three repetitions of spoken text can cause listeners to describe speech as song. In hearing a spoken phrase repeatedly, we tend to focus on the melodic features: the more strongly melodic the phrase (wide pitch patterns, for example), the more likely we are to hear it as 'sung' when it repeats. However, the illusion does not depend solely on repetition. Properties of the language we hear and our competence in that language can affect whether we perceive a repeated spoken phrase as song. Speech appears more song-like if our language is non-tonal, if we do not understand the language and if we perceive the language as 'difficult' to pronounce. For example, if we have no experience in a tonal language such as Mandarin, we may not be sure if we are listening to someone talking or singing (Deutsch, 2010).

These experiments raise questions about how people with perceptual and linguistic differences hear and perceive songs – do they perceive speech as more song-like until they develop a certain level of language knowledge? Which aspects of speech or song do they focus on? I do not have clear answers to these questions, but the boundaries between speech and song are not fixed; it is possible that some children and some adults do not perceive speech and song as separate acts. This gives us greater scope for using singing to support, develop, supplement or even replace speech. We do know that singing can be easier to *process* than speech. This is because singing, like infant-directed speech, can emphasize aspects of speech and voice, making it easier to perceive speech sounds, words and phrases (see Chapter 3).

Additionally, like infant-directed speech, singing uses the brain's right hemisphere more than it does the left hemisphere. When we process verbal communication, most of us process temporal aspects (rhythm, changes over time) in the left hemisphere of our brain and spectral information (pitch, timbre, tone) in our right hemisphere. Although both song and speech activate both brain hemispheres, 'speech' relies more on left-hemisphere processing and 'song' on the right hemisphere. When adult English speakers process speech efficiently, they show strong activation in the anterior (front) left hemisphere. However, people with *autism* and *Down syndrome* show subtle differences (Groen, Alku & Bishop, 2008; Welsh, Elliott & Simon, 2003; Pearson & Hodgetts, 2020). Although they process music and song in both hemispheres in the same way as their neurotypical peers, they show weaker processing in their left hemisphere. Weaker processing in the left hemisphere for speech is linked to increased language difficulties in *autism*, *Down syndrome* and *dyslexia* (see Cowell, 2010). Weak left-hemisphere processing is also found in English speakers when they listen to a tonal language such as Mandarin and cannot be certain if they hear song or speech (Deutsch, 2010). Therefore, there can be a part of the speech-song spectrum that is ambiguous for all of us. Some children and young adults whose brains are organized or process language differently might respond more strongly to singing or to strongly melodic speech than to adult-directed speech.

This discussion raises the question of whether we could or should use more of a singing style of speech with some people at the early stages of verbal learning. We tend to use adult-directed speech with older children and adults because we do not wish to seem condescending or have not considered singing instead. An exaggerated form of speech might have advantages similar to song – song-like speech may assist processing and increase focus and attention on verbal communication. For example, research by Dr Rosemary Ridgway (2013) showed that in comparison to speech, singing helped children with profound and multiple learning difficulties become more comfortable with close social contact. When the children were being sung to, they were more attentive, more tolerant of social proximity and responded with more facial and physical expressions of pleasure. For some children and adults who are at early levels of communication, song may remain more appealing than speech.

Songs and singing-based communication might make it easier for some learners to focus on speech sounds and attend to and enjoy verbal communication. Once we have engaged learners, we can use songs and singing activities to encourage vocal and verbal production, and to teach words and phrases. In his *Tuning In Music Book*, Adam Ockelford (2018) gives examples of 'micro-songs', which teach short, functional phrases using short songs with distinct rhythmic and melodic patterns. These patterns echo those of speech but exaggerate them a little: this draws on the principles we use for infant-directed speech but offers structure and routine. These micro-songs provide learners with an expressive form of language midway between speech and song. We will return to this principle later when we consider the possibility of skills transferring from song to speech.

Once learners are practising using words through song, we can use singing and songs to develop the skills that underpin speech intelligibility.

How can singing support speech intelligibility?

The term 'intelligibility' refers to how another person speaks so that we can understand them. We can have difficulty understanding someone's speech for many reasons, including our difficulty in 'calibrating' some of the individualistic ways someone might speak. However, some people can have speech that remains hard to understand, even to people who know them well. The causes of poor speech intelligibility are linked to multiple factors, including unclear articulation of speech sounds, or unusual use of pitch, stress or speech rhythm. Some of these skills can be developed through singing. The skills we enhance through singing are likely to transfer to speech. This is because singing uses the same over-lapping neurological networks (the O of OPERA – Patel, 2011, 2014, see Chapter 1) and muscles as voice and speech and because singing requires a greater level of *precision* and control over the voice and speech muscles (P), and *attention* to pitch and tone (A). Compared to talking, songs and singing can be a more *engaging* (E) way to learn and afford more opportunities for learners to *repeat* with precision (R). Furthermore, we might not need to help learners improve every aspect of intelligibility. Articulation, fluency and intonation each contribute to the intelligibility of speech and a slight improvement in any of these can help learners make themselves understood more easily. Minor differences can accu-mulate over time to have more significant effects, especially if changes are made when young. We will look, below, at each skill in turn.

Intelligible speech relies partly on *articulation*. To articulate a sound, we need fine control over our voice and articulators (tongue, lips, soft palate). It can take at least five years to master the fine motor skills needed for speech sounds. It can take much longer to master sounds in words and combine articulatory precision with prosody (rhythm and melody). For some children and young people, some speech sounds will remain undeveloped into adulthood. Even then, the complex motor, cognitive and sensory systems that we use when we speak can come under stress, causing well-rehearsed sounds or words to falter. We might experience this ourselves in moments of high cognitive load; for exam-ple, a demanding task or a state of heightened emotion can provoke hesitations, stammering, false starts or spoonerisms (see also Chapter 3, and Video 2 in the online resources).

Singing can be an effective way to develop articulation and to prac-tise producing sounds in speech. For example, you could work with a speech and language therapist to identify which speech sounds a learner should work on. You could select songs and singing activities that allow the learner to repeat target sounds in initial, medial, final position, and in diverse words. You can vary the singing tempo to encourage skills that support clear articulation. Slow, exaggerated miming to songs, for example, can help support somatosensory feedback for speech sounds, whereas we can promote faster movements of target sounds if we speed up.

Singing can support *fluent speech*. Most songs have a defined beat. As we have seen (Chapter 3), a beat can reduce stuttering by supporting motor planning. A song has a rhythmic structure that aligns with the beat of songs, and this can help children plan and produce articula-tory movements of words. Therefore, singing a song can help learners make sounds and words with greater ease and fluency. We can also use rhythmic priming to enhance production. As discussed in Chapter 6, rhythmic priming helps us perceive the durational contrasts and pat-terns in words and phrases. Priming can prepare the brain for speaking and help us control the subtle changes in volume, pitch and duration that accentuate syllables or words in phrases. We can teach the rhythmic patterns of phrases in songs to support fluency; this will also encourage musicality. We can also reduce the articulatory demands by singing on syllables or simple consonant-vowel combinations. For example, a learner could sing and intone speech-based phrases using vowels to capture the rhythm and pitch. Such small changes can slowly build the skills and motor processes that support intelligible speech production while reducing cognitive load and stress.

Intonation in speech refers to the rise and fall of our voice and how we use our vocal range. Intonation contributes to intelligibility, as it can clarify our intent or meaning. In spoken English, contrasting intonation can differentiate a question (rising pitch) from a statement of fact (falling pitch). The range of our voice as we speak communicates whether we are feeling excited, neutral or underwhelmed. Because intonation relies on control of the vocal folds, it can be a difficult skill for some learn-ers with motor difficulties or weaknesses, such as those with *cerebral palsy*, *dyspraxia* or *Down syndrome*. People who have weak muscles for breathing, phonation or articulation can have difficulties controlling the vocal intensity, pitch and volume (see Chapters 7 and 8). These types of problems can interfere with clear communication. For example, some people with Down syndrome use a smaller vocal range when speaking and tend to use fewer inflexions. They might use less clear pitch changes to mark the end of spoken phrases and signal questions, affecting how easily they communicate meaning and emotion (but see Rachel, Figure 4.1, and listen to an example in Video 3 in the online resources). People with *autism* can also have difficulties in using appropriate intonation in speech. They often have superior skills in processing melody in non-speech but can struggle to tell the difference between questions and statements.

Singing songs can help young people practise using changes in pitch, and vocal warm-ups and exercises can help prepare the voice for using the entire vocal range. Songs and singing activities can also teach the melodic shape of target words and phrases we would like learners to speak. For example, micro-songs can help children learn functional phrases, such as 'yes, please', 'more', 'no, thank you'. The *Tuning In* book and cards (Ockelford, 2018) and the Amber Trust website give examples of songs that can support learners in understanding simple phrases: each short phrase has its own melodic line to support comprehension. These can be a proxy for the words. For example, a non-verbal learner might hum the tune to communicate the words (see also Way to Play, Chapter 5). Likewise, we might use a pitched instrument rather than a voice to support the perception of intonational contours in speech. The vocal signal is complex and can be challenging to process. We should remember that some do not wish to use their voice to communicate. Focusing on intonational patterns through music offers an alternative way to express simple phrases.

Case study: Singing and intelligibility

Meg is a keen singer who has severe hearing loss. Her poor hearing acuity affects the quality of feedback she receives from her ears and via bone conduction when she sings and speaks. As a result, her speech lacks definition. When talking, she relies on a limited range of conso-nants and vowels: her repertoire is limited to sounds that she can see, such as /m/, /b/, /sh/ and /s/. Her voice is soft, and there is minimal variation in rhythm or pitch when she speaks and sings. Meg also has Down syndrome; she has poorly coordinated and weak oro-motor movements and some broader motor coordination and planning difficulties. For example, although she can perceive and produce the speech sounds /p/, /t/ and /k/ in isolation, she cannot make these as a sequence of sounds. This can indicate a motor planning difficulty.

Because of her hearing loss and weak auditory memory, Meg struggles to learn new songs, especially when working in a group. However, she made incredible progress over just six weeks, with some minor adaptations. If I positioned her in the group to see my mouth movements when singing, she could more easily perceive the sounds and did not need to work so hard to filter out other noises and people. Like other people with hearing loss, she could perceive rhythm better than the melody. To make it easier for Meg to sense the rhythms including clapping, hand gestures and graphic scores. I drew the melodic shape of songs in the air with my hand, then drew their lines on paper. I provided pictures representing recurring words in songs to support her auditory memory and knowledge of target sounds; later, Makaton gestures were enough to prompt recall of these. Once Meg had visual support and prompts, she grew in confidence and mastered the unfamiliar elements of the song. When I compared the songs she sang in week six to her first performances in weeks one and two, she progressed in pitching, melodic shape, rhythm and articulation. In just six weeks, Meg had reproduced:

- the melodic shape with a broader vocal range
- intervals of a third
- some speech sounds that repeated within the song
- some target speech sounds consistently
- clear contrasts of duration in long and short syllables.

The example of Meg illustrates how quickly singing can support speech, even in someone with complex, long-standing needs. I had seen these types of changes before, when I examined the effects of singing on intelligibility in a group of singers, compared to a control group. Like Meg, the singers showed modest improvements in different aspects of voice and speech: when I compared the changes to those in the control group, some changes were statistically significant, indicating that the singing programme caused the changes. Each learner was 20 years old and had been receiving speech therapy regularly for two to three years. These minor changes could have snowballed if they were younger when we initiated these activities.

HOW DO I SUPPORT SONG LEARNING?

When learning songs, neurotypical children can make poor progress because of under-matured motor systems or poor feedback about accuracy in pitch, articulation and timing. Children and adults in neurodiverse groups will face similar difficulties. Their progress may also be affected by differences in cognitive, conceptual, physiological or sensory systems. We can adapt how we teach to reduce the effects of some difficulties that limit singing potential. In doing so, we can help the young person develop their skills in perceiving speech and reproducing words and phrases. The sections below discuss how memory, cognitive load and sensory and conceptual differences can affect the learning of songs.

Different trajectories: auditory-verbal memory and cognitive load

In Chapter 5, we examined how performing multiple motor activities could reduce performance in rhythmic motor tasks. We can think of singing as a dual motor task, too. When we sing, we need to plan and coordinate our oral and laryngeal systems with our breath, and monitor our timing and our pitching – either against an internal template of a song's key or against an external cue, such as another singer, a backing track, or similar. At the same time, we might want to recall the meaning of words and their sounds. Singing songs is, therefore, a demanding process, cognitively and physiologically. Learning to sing new songs is especially demanding of our working memory because we learn songs by listening and repeating what we hear. Using our working memory while performing another task can cause excessive 'cognitive load'. Our performance deteriorates when the task demands overload our attention, memory and motor control. If we are under cognitive load while speaking, we place our speech and vocal systems under stress. This affects our voice quality, and we might begin to stutter, hesitate or omit speech sounds.

The processes of verbal imitation and speech planning can increase cognitive load in people who have difficulty processing sounds, such as those with auditory processing demands, hearing loss or limited auditory-verbal memory. Until they have learned the words of a song, they might have more difficulty than usual when singing or reproducing sounds or words. For many children and young people, simplifying the task or reducing the demands on working memory makes it easier to use their voice. Some, such as Rachel, below, and Figure 4.1, might automatically simplify the task to make the process easier.

Case study: Rachel: The problem with consonants

Rachel has a musical way of speaking and singing. She is very good at reproducing the melodic shape of songs and the rhythm structure of words – but she omits speech sounds, syllables and melodic intervals. There are differences in how the brains of people with Down syndrome process speech, and these might help explain why Rachel finds it easy to sing melody, but hard to sing words.

Most people with Down syndrome tend to reproduce the gist of something rather than the detail. Rachel's ability to produce the 'big' prosodic features of song and speech reflects this global processing style. In addition, speech and articulation are hard work for people with Down syndrome due to weaker muscles and hypermobility that inhibit the precise formation of sounds and coordination with voice. For these reasons, Rachel probably finds it easier to reproduce the melody and vowel sounds, which require less precise motor move- ments than consonants and intervals.

There may also be a difference in how Rachel's brain processes songs and words. When we learn songs, there is evidence that vowels are strongly connected to the melody and processed in the right hemisphere. In contrast, we process consonants separately in the left hemisphere, which is a weaker hemisphere in people with Down syndrome (Kolinsky et al., 2009; Lidji et al., 2010). If our brains divide words in songs into consonants and vowels, and store these in separate neural systems, we must retrieve both sets of information when we want to sing. Rachel might have greater difficulty than peers in retrieving the consonants from her left hemisphere. If she tries to recall the consonants, this will increase cognitive load, leading to more speech errors, a higher rate of sounds being missed out and difficulty in using the voice. In comparison, retrieving the melody and vowels only is relatively easy, as these are processed together in her stronger right hemisphere. In other words, Rachel may have extra difficulty processing or producing speech sounds in situations requiring multiple processing, for example speech sounds and rhythm, and melody and meaning.

The case study of Rachel above shows how multiple cognitive, phys-iological, perceptual and syndrome-specific factors can change *how* a song is learned. Most children and adults seem to spontaneously reduce their processing load when learning a new song by limiting production to words and the overall 'shape' of the song. With repetition, they add increasing rhythmic and melodic detail to the output. Like Meg, Rachel seems to have difficulty mastering the words in songs. However, if we break down and simplify the task of learning a song, we can help Rachel, and others, learn songs more quickly and accurately. For example, we can ask Rachel to sing the song using a simple vowel sound. This will help her process the melodic shape (melody and rhythm) without over-loading her memory, thus reducing cognitive load and improving vocal accuracy. Rachel could then listen to the words as they are sung – as speech production is slower in song than speech, this can support the processing of speech sounds. Deconstructing the task would reduce the cognitive demands of first learning the words.

Once the global elements of the song are in place, Rachel may more readily attend to phonetic details. People with Down syndrome can develop stable representations of speech sounds with sufficient exposure (Gathercole, 2006). However, Rachel would need encouragement to practise speech segments, words and motor tasks slowly and accurately during the learning process. Accurate and 'error-free' rehearsal can reduce the effort associated with whole-word production in people with apraxia of speech – a focus on precision when learning can support the automatic production of words (Whiteside *et al.*, 2012). For Rachel, a similar strategy during word-learning tasks could reduce the cognitive load for speech production.

SUPPORTING SINGING AND SONG-LEARNING IN LEARNERS WITH ADDITIONAL NEEDS

The final sections of this chapter consider how to set up favourable con-ditions that can help young people use and learn words through songs and singing activities. I do not explain how to support singing skills and technique; instead, I explain how you can use musical activities to encourage vocal expression, how to practise speech sounds for songs to support articulation and phonation, and how to reduce the nega-tive effects of cognitive load during song-learning. There are example activities in the online resources, and useful books and websites in the 'Recommended reading and resources' section.

General principles for supporting singing development

Below are some general principles we can use to help learners of any age with singing. These principles are derived from the stages we all go through when learning to sing. We can also use these stages to highlight issues we might need to consider for learners with different developmental pathways. In particular:

- Start from the developmental level of the singer (e.g. Welch, 1998; Rutkowski, 1997), rather than their age. Singing skills will develop broadly in line with motor maturity. However, some children and adults with motor differences might remain at an earlier developmental level, depending on their unique needs.
- Experiment with vocal play. Singing is physical. We need to learn to coordinate the various muscle groups, as we saw in Chapter 7. Playing with vocal and verbal sound can help develop the different muscles and support control over pitch and rhythm.
- Look for different learning patterns. Most young children find it easier to learn the words than melodies; their singing progresses from 'speech-like chanting' towards a more melodic and expressive form of song. However, some learners might follow a different path, especially if they have difficulties hearing, perceiving, remembering or producing words.
- Support melodic contour before 'filling in' detail. Melodic contour develops before discrete pitches and intervals. It may be easier to reproduce melodic shape and intervals on vowels or single syllables than words.
- Consider the singer's cultural background: the music they hear and their language may use different tonal systems and rhythmic patterns.
- Choose songs with intervals that develop first or are represented well in infant-directed speech. Intervals of thirds and fifths may be easier to master when learning to sing. This is partly because of enculturation and partly as a result of maturation.
- Work within the young person's existing vocal range. When learning, children sing best within their usual speaking range. Children develop a wider pitch range as they mature, gain

experience and develop motor control. It may be possible to develop the range gradually through gentle practice.

- Singing tends to be more accurate if the singer can hear themselves – group singing can reduce accuracy. It also improves if the learner can see the singer's face, especially their mouth. We might consider small groups or one-to-one tuition for younger singers or people with altered sensory perception or hearing loss.
- Reduce task demands during learning to reduce the effects of cognitive load. Song learning is more accessible if the task is broken down into phrases. You could provide lyrics (if the child/adult can read) and other cues to teach and prompt words.
- Be specific in the feedback you give learners. Feedback helps us know what we might need to adjust (e.g. pitching, tone, posture). Visual feedback can help us to help ourselves – a simple guitar tuner or singing app can show us if we are close to the correct pitch, and apps or software (such as the free software, *Praat*) can show spectrographic information to help us adjust tone and resonance.

These principles can help us notice how a learner is developing and alert us to possible differences in learning trajectories. I will discuss adaptation to address specific differences in learning below.

Strategies to encourage vocal and verbal communication

Our primary focus in this book is speech. Still, we can use songs, singing and musical activities with pre-verbal learners or those who prefer alternative means of communication.

- Use recorders, whistles and kazoos instead of voice. These instruments can be the first step towards spoken sounds for reluctant singers. You can use them to emulate rhythms in words and practise breathing for vocalizing. Once the child has begun to vocalize, you can progress from recorders to kazoos. They also provide essential sensory-based training (see Berger, 2015 for detailed examples).
- Use songs that students can lead, so that they can take part without words. You can use props, such as scarves, puppets, toys, written words and visual images, so that they can select

the songs. For example, they can choose coloured scarves for a group of learners to 'sing'.

- Encourage turn-taking by letting young people complete the end of sentences in songs in any way they choose – a look, a gesture, a shake of an instrument.
- Use songs and games where students can choose a specific word or phrase to be sung; for example, they might substitute their name or those of their friends, family, pets or toys in songs they know well. 'He's got the whole world in his hands' was a favourite song for this, among my groups; they would substitute 'the whole world' with their own noun.
- In emerging singers, use a microphone to increase volume and auditory feedback; this can work with vocal learners to discourage excessive use of tension when singing.
- Use a microphone with sound effects to encourage vocal experimentation and attention to sound.
- Use resonators that respond well to voices (e.g. drums, stringed instruments) so that learners can hear their voice in them, or feel them vibrate in sympathy.
- Use SOVT activities with straws in water so learners use their voice and can see it move the water, without worrying about hearing it. This can encourage young people who are anxious about singing, and encourage phonation without strain.
- Encourage young people to become aware of how their voice feels (e.g. place fingers to the voice box while singing).
- Use a visual representation of own voice – some apps use spectrograms that show voice in real-time (e.g. *Praat*) and can show pitching accuracy. This can encourage learners to use a wider range, to develop pitching accuracy and to play with resonance and timbre.
- Let learners draw vocal patterns to sing using pens, gestures – or even toys. Cars can 'drive' up and down melodic lines that you draw, puppets can 'sing' the patterns, finger-puppet bumblebees can 'humm' and fly pitch glides and swoops.

Use warm-ups to support articulation and voice

Traditional vocal warm-up exercises can be adapted to help young people develop specific sounds; you can sing scales and arpeggios on any words that are suitable. You can create bespoke routines that use 'total' communication, including cued articulation, colourful semantics, visual and signed representations of key words, and video-modelling of articulatory movements (Lindley-Baker & Mills, 2022). You can also use any song to encourage articulation. Choose a song the group likes and perform different exercises along to it before singing together:

- Whisper or mouth words to songs as a warm-up to support articulatory movements. This will minimize the processing demands associated with word recall and oro-motor coordination.
- Sing vowels or neutral syllables ('loo') to songs/choruses to encourage sustained phonation and articulation, while minimizing processing demands.
- Use /mm/ or /ng/ sounds to support sensation of voice and movement of the soft palate. You can also use kazoos to encourage easy phonation – again, without the cognitive load of using words.

Support attention and processing during learning

Even though singing can be less effortful than speech, we can still easily overload the system if we expect everything – voice, breath, melody, articulation – to come together. We must be mindful of developing precision (the P in OPERA) in any skills we hope will transfer, and ultimately this means we should aim for error-free production. Still, we must balance this drive for precision with E for emotional engagement and A for attention. That might mean that we use very short, targeted singing activities to focus on building foundational skills in singing, and then we let go: give them a microphone and let them sing. We need to make singing as easy as possible to reduce cognitive load. We also need to ensure that the learner can see, feel, hear or otherwise sense when they are doing it right. In practice, then, we might use the following strategies:

- Offer physiological support – such as splints or Kinesio tape – to support postural stability and increase proprioception; some young people might need to sing while seated, rather than standing, to reduce vestibular-postural demands, or to sing against a floor, resonance board or wall to increase somatosensory sensations.
- Reduce demands on auditory memory – teach phrases for songs one at a time: use rhythmic priming by clapping rhythms of the

words and phrase before singing them (see Chapter 8); provide images, Makaton or actions to symbolize and prompt the word learning and recall; use vowels, rather than words, when learning the melodic shape of the phrase.

- Reduce processing demands – for example, focus on 'good' phonation separately from articulation. Aim for good tone across a phrase, using a vowel or neutral syllable, humming or /ng/ – ask the learner to listen to or 'think the words' as they do this. Once established, focus on maintaining posture on the out-breath, so the last sound is as clear as the first sound – break the phrase into shorter phrases if necessary. You could learn part of the song using sign language or create your own actions to represent words. This can support word recall without using voice; later, use the signs to support the young people as they sing.

- Use very short, targeted singing activities to focus on building foundational skills. Alternate periods of focused practice with relaxed 'fun' sessions. Leave time between practice: we all learn songs gradually and our brains need time to 'build' the foundation between practice sessions. Too much repetition and new learning in the same session can interfere with this process (Katz, Ando & Wiseheart, 2021).

CAN SKILLS TRANSFER FROM SONGS TO SPONTANEOUS SPEECH?

If we do all we can to support learners when learning a song, will they be able to use the words and phrases they learn in a song for everyday conversation? This is the big question, and in the Introduction to this book, I suggested we remain cautious about this. However, the example below shows that skills learned in singing can transfer spontaneously. Kerry was one of my PhD participants (Jeffery, 2016). To my surprise, when I asked her to speak the words of 'Happy Birthday', she did so with remarkable ease.

Case study: Happy Birthday

Kerry fought to speak. A stutter caused her words to stick in her throat. When it broke free, her voice sounded harsh, jagged and low-pitched. You could hear and see the physical and cognitive effort it took just for her to say hello. However, singing was easy for Kerry. Her voice was softer and flowed without difficulty over an octave's range.

Singing revealed Kerry's talent for matching pitches and tunes. She learned new songs quickly: she reproduced the melodic shape after listening once, then began to learn the words and the intervals. However, mastering the words came at a cost. She lost pitching accuracy when singing lyrics, and her voice would falter as she struggled to recall words. It was clear that strategies to reduce the strain on her auditory-verbal memory would help her as she was learning to sing new songs; we could later 'stretch' her abilities by introducing dual attention and dual motor tasks.

As singing came easily to Kerry, compared to speaking, I wondered if she could speak the words of songs she knew well. I asked her to sing and then speak Happy Birthday. Kerry sang the song melodically – she produced well-tuned melodic intervals and she kept within key. Her rhythmic timing was also good; it was disrupted once, when she paused to work out who to sing Happy Birthday to. However, the surprise came when Kerry spoke the words. Kerry did not stutter as she spoke the song, and her voice quality was close to modal. She spoke the words with a wide pitch range and a clear pulse and rhythm. Her previous experience of singing the song directly influenced how she spoke it. In turn, this gave her better access to her own speech and voice.

It is not surprising that Kerry's speech was fluent when singing: the beat and rhythm of songs are known to promote fluency, as we discussed in Chapter 5. Singing words enables the formation of internal timing cues for speech, reducing stuttering (Alm, 2004), which improves phonation (Ludlow & Loucks, 2003; Salihovíc et al., 2009). However, it was a surprise that she remained fluent when speaking the words, and that she found it easy to use her voice when speaking the song. Why might this be? I identified three possible explanations:

1. Possibly, the task reduced her cognitive load. For Kerry, speaking the song did not overload her working memory like conversational speech, as she needed to *recall* rather than *formulate*. She recalled each phrase as a single unit, along with the rhythmic motor plan for its prosody and speech sounds (see Chapter 3).
2. Learning to sing words rather than speaking them might be a

better fit for Kerry's brain. Brain scans have shown that the control of speech movements when singing text, rather than saying the same words, occurs in the right hemisphere (Jeffries, Fritz & Braun, 2003), which, as we have seen, is stronger in people with Down syndrome.

3. Singing words places greater demands on the cerebellar circuitry than speaking the words, and assists motor timing for oral articulation and control of the larynx and phonation (Jeffries *et al.*, 2003). Some researchers believe this is why singing can help speech (Wan *et al.*, 2010).

Therefore, for Kerry, learning to produce words while singing may assist speech production by laying down appropriate motor memory and reducing cognitive load while enhancing aspects of precision in motor timing within the brain. This sets up favourable conditions for fluency, phonation and potential transfer between domains.

Kerry had difficulty speaking some phrases, even though they were probably well learned. Her second and third spoken phrases of the song were different from the first phrase in terms of rhythm, fluency and phonation. Phrase three was naturalistic in rhythm and melody, but phrase four was initially dysfluent with lengthy pauses between each word, and her voice quality became harsher. We all tend to find it harder to recall lines of a song or poem after the first line; experiments with adults show that when we recall song lyrics, we do this based on 'lines' or grouped phrases, and memory for words is strongest for the initial lines (Racette & Peretz, 2007).

What can we learn from Kerry about transfer?

The transference of song lyrics to speech can place higher demands on *working memory* and *attention* (*cognitive load*) than singing. Transferring lyrics to speech will be challenging for people who have weaknesses in verbal memory or working memory, or who have problems with sustaining or dividing attention, serial recall and sequencing of verbal information. However, these are the skills that we must develop if we wish skills to transfer between domains. Despite the challenge that Kerry faced when asked to separate the words from the melody (Racette & Peretz, 2007), her speech and voice improved – and this happened for other participants in my research. If we can support learners to practise words fluently in the context of singing, it allows them to develop and practise motor plans for speech. This may ultimately reduce the planning load for speech production. This example of spontaneous transfer shows that skills *can* transfer, and that the transference may free up vocal and articulatory abilities. If we make the process deliberate, we can discover the long-term impacts for learners like Kerry, especially if we begin supporting musical skills for speech from a young age.

CHAPTER SUMMARY

Singing can be easier to process than speech: its characteristics aid language learning and perception of words from infancy. Singing is processed in the right hemisphere of the brain, which can be more efficient for some learners than the language-dominant left hemisphere. Singing offers slower production and emphasizes speech sounds. Its rhythmic component helps carry and focus attention and supports fluency and motor skills planning. For all we know, singing may continue to offer these benefits in older children and adults who might not differentiate between singing and speech. Singing can therefore be a more powerful means of supporting the perception of speech sounds than adult-directed speech. Learners with hearing loss can benefit from what singing can offer: although noticeable changes may be small, they reflect improved representations of words and more stable motor production. With time, singing can strengthen articulation and vocal control and can be used to practise words and phrases for speech. However, we must also be mindful of the limitations. We need to be careful to balance training for speech against enjoyment and individuality and to consider what skills are worth prioritizing. Singing places additional demands and control on our speech systems, strengthening the physiological and motoric responses, but these systems are easily upset when processing demands become too high. For this reason, benefits may not readily transfer to conversational speech, which places additional stresses on our cognitive and verbal systems. We will examine this more in the next chapter. Meanwhile, singing and singing games offer plenty to encourage developing musical and speaking skills, even for pre-verbal learners or those who prefer not to speak.

RECOMMENDED READING AND RESOURCES
Singing pedagogy and voice

Fisher, J. & Kayes, G. (2018). *This Is a Voice: 99 Exercises to Train, Project, and Harness the Power of Your Voice*. London: Wellcome Collection.

Loney, N. & Adams, M. (2018). *Vocal Warm-ups and Technical Exercises for Kids*. Hemford, Ontario: Full Voice Music.

Phillips, K. (1996). *Teaching Kids to Sing*. New York, NY: Schirmer.

Williams, J. (2018). *Teaching Singing to Children and Young Adults* (second edition). Abingdon, Oxfordshire: Compton Publishing.

Singing development

Houlahan, M. & Tacka, P. (2015). *Kodály Today: A Cognitive Approach to Elementary Music Education*. Oxford: Oxford University Press.

Welch, G.F. (2015). Singing and Vocal Development. In G. McPherson (ed.), *The Child as Musician: A Handbook of Musical Development*. Oxford: Oxford University Press.

Songs and communication activities for people with complex needs

The Amber Trust and Amber Plus website – musical resources to help families and practitioners who work with young people with profound and multiple learning difficulties. It includes songs, musical activities and apps https://amberplus.ambertrust.org.

Lloyd, P. (2007). *Let's All Listen. Songs for Group Work in Settings that Include Students with Learning Difficulties and Autism*. London: Jessica Kingsley Publishers.

Ockelford, A. (2018). *Tuning In Music Book: Sixty-Four Songs for Children with Complex Needs and Visual Impairment to Promote Language, Social Interaction and Wider Development*. London: Jessica Kingsley Publishers.

PART 3

Conclusion

CHAPTER 10

Making Music Work for Speech and Wellbeing

THE BIG QUESTIONS

How do we support someone's musical skills to help new skills transfer to the spoken domain? At the same time, how do we maintain enjoyment and exploit the power of music to promote wellbeing?

By the end of this chapter, you will:

- know why we need to focus on attention to support the transfer of skills from music to speech
- understand how 'flow' can support engagement for learning and wellbeing – and why this matters for transfer
- be able to adapt an activity to meet multiple objectives, including musical precision, engagement, attention and enjoyment.

WHO IS THIS FOR?

This chapter applies to all children and young people. It explains how we can support enjoyment while also encouraging musical development.

Previous chapters have explored the barriers children and young people might face when developing verbal and musical skills. We have considered how we can adapt activities to support learning in people with sensory, physical, cognitive and developmental needs. The big questions that remain are: how do we help a child or young adult develop their musical skills so that new music-based skills transfer to the spoken domain; at the same time, how do we help them enjoy making music, and how can these activities support their wellbeing?

This chapter gives examples of how you can structure learning activities to meet an individual's learning needs and align with the conditions that support transfer. We will revisit the OPERA (Patel, 2011, 2014) and PRISM (Fiveash *et al.*, 2021) theories and examine why attention is critical to transfer. I compare these theories with the principles of 'flow' (Csikszentmihalyi, 1990). We can apply these theories to help learners enjoy their learning and increase the likelihood that their skills will transfer from music to speech.

USING MUSIC SKILLS FOR LEARNING: HOW DO WE BEST SUPPORT LEARNERS?

Now that we understand more about the skills of our learners in musical and verbal domains, we will revisit the conditions that are required to support the transfer from music to speech. The OPERA hypothesis (Patel, 2011, see Chapter 1) explained what requirements are needed for learning to transfer between music and language domains: Overlap (in areas of the brain); Precision (in music-making); Emotion (connection and enjoyment with the music); Repetition (of learning); Attention (to sound and performance). When a learner is fully engaged and repeatedly using musical skills to a higher degree of precision than needed for speech, their learning will likely transfer from music to language. There is some debate about whether – or how much – difference music training can make to language (e.g. Jentschke, 2016; Wisniewski, Mantell & Pfordresher, 2013) because we do not yet fully understand how much 'overlap' there is between music and language systems in the brain, or how early experiences, developmental trajectories and genetics affect the transfer. However, the transfer of related or 'near-transfer' skills is more widely accepted (Miendlarzewska & Trost, 2014). For example, most researchers acknowledge that music-making activities support listening and sensory-motor integration because music uses these skills. Likewise, they agree music supports phonological processing because both music training and phonological processing require us to notice and process rhythmic changes in sound. Skills developed in singing should benefit speech (Patel, 2011, 2014). These draw on the same physiological processes, and at least some of the same neurological networks, so skills learned through singing are 'within domain' and do not need to transfer.

Additionally, learners with significant language needs might benefit more from music than learners with more advanced verbal skills (Swaminathan & Schellenberg, 2020). However, minimal research examines how theories such as OPERA and PRISM apply to learners with multiple or complex needs or developmental delays. Although there is considerable potential for these learners to benefit from making music, we might have to work harder to support the skills needed for transfer. Later in this chapter, we will examine ways to manage this.

If we wish to exploit the full potential of music-making for verbal learning, we must understand a little more about each of the five conditions that support the transfer of skills from the music domain to the language domain; we must also consider how we address these conditions when working with learners. We will revisit each condition of OPERA below and evaluate the implication of working with learners who are on different developmental pathways.

OPERA revisited

OVERLAP

This condition states that music must engage the same anatomical or brain networks that we need for language. Unless we know otherwise, we must assume that our learners use the same neural networks and systems when making music as children with less complex needs. Previous chapters have considered how skills such as beat entrainment (Chapter 2), rhythm perception and production (Chapters 3 and 4) overlap with the brain processes and cognitive skills needed for spoken language. We have considered the physiological similarities and differences between speech and song: the overlap exists at many levels. It is taken for granted (Patel, 2014) that transfer between song and speech will occur. Music sessions that use songs as teaching activities will probably have more immediate benefits for speech than sessions based on non-verbal music. However, we should incorporate non-verbal rhythm training, too. These skills provide a foundation for musicality, as well as verbal learning.

PRECISION

For the transfer between domains to occur, the child or adult must play or sing with greater accuracy than needed for speech: this makes the overlapping brain regions work much harder than they need to for speech. Previous chapters suggested how to help learners become more precise in beat, rhythm and singing. However, some people will have lifelong difficulties producing or synchronizing movements despite adaptations. For example, the brain networks that control limbs, voice and articulation can be damaged in people with neuromuscular conditions such as cerebral palsy. Brain damage and weak or stiff muscles can impede motor timing and accuracy, even if we adjust tempo to their 'best' tempo. Music-making can help the brain improve multisensory coordination and motor timing in people with cerebral palsy and other motor difficulties (e.g. Thaut, 2005). However, we cannot predict how soon an individual will benefit from such changes or how much. But even if accuracy in timing remains a challenge, the attempt to match movements may enhance beat perception – attempting to entrain requires the learner to listen to sound in a focused, active style, which is critical for speech perception. Additionally, the rhythmicity of music can make motor movements easier to produce (e.g. see Thaut, 2005). Greater physical ease when moving will increase the chances of entraining with precision.

EMOTION

The child or adult must be emotionally engaged and enjoy the activity before learning transfers. For most learners, music-making is rewarding, and playing music can release 'feel-good' chemicals (Levitin, 2019) that encourage participation. However, there is potential tension between the need to maintain an emotional (E) connection with the activity while also playing with precision (P) and attention (A, below). If we focus on accuracy too much or for too long, the learner may become bored, anxious or stressed, affecting their enjoyment and ability to attend. We need to keep focused (precise) practice short, even if this potentially slows the rate of progress.

REPETITION

We must repeat musical activities. Focused practice is needed to develop the 'right' neural pathways in the brain and encourage transfer to speech. Through repetition, the neuronal connections are strengthened and regional areas of the brain adapt and grow. However, repetition can be tedious and counter-productive. We can teach the same skill in different ways to maintain interest. Still, we also need to plan for frequency and duration of practice – regular, short periods of focused training are better for our brains than more prolonged periods of practice.

ATTENTION

The musical activities we use must engage the attentional areas of the brain. This may be the most challenging condition to meet. As we have seen (Chapters 2 and 3), as children, our abilities to attend to different aspects of rhythm develop quite slowly (Drake *et al.,* 2000). Furthermore, the brain regions that support advanced attentional skills are not fully matured until we reach our twenties (Sousa, 2016). We need to plan how best to support attention in young people whose brains develop more slowly or who process information differently. We must help them practise advanced attention skills, such as focused attention, sustained attention, attentional switching and inhibition. We might need to modify the environment to help them with this; the fewer distractions, the better.

ADDITIONAL CONSIDERATIONS FROM THEORY: ATTENTION AND ADAPTATION SKILLS
Cognition, attention and executive functions

In 2014, Patel updated the OPERA theory (Patel, 2014) to incorporate evidence from neuroscientists who examined the cognitive processes of music-to-language transfer (e.g. Besson *et al.,* 2011). The revised OPERA theory emphasizes the role of cognition in the transfer of learning from music to speech. Specifically, it emphasises that music activities must 'stretch' auditory attention and auditory memory. The music psychologist, Franziska Degé (2021), expounded on this. According to Degé, we are working intensively with the core components of language when we make music: she said we are 'doing' auditory discrimination, memorizing passages of sound, learning to recognize patterns in structure, training motor movements, coordination and timing. Degé argues that music may be more efficient than other activities – such as sport – in developing these executive functions. Making music requires 'higher-order' executive function skills, including self-monitoring, practising with discipline, inhibiting competing motor impulses and switching between tasks/activities. These higher-order skills have clear links with OPERA (e.g. precision, attention) and may be why so many trained musicians perform better than non-musicians in skills that underpin learning.

Many of the adaptations and strategies that I have suggested in previous chapters aim to enhance attention by reducing the demands placed on auditory memory to offset cognitive load and associated emotional stress. But by reducing the demands on a learner's working memory, are we setting up conditions for transfer to fail? Not necessarily. Patel argues that instrumental music places higher demands on auditory working memory than speech because we cannot use word meaning: we must store the sounds and sequence without any other 'tags' to help us. Even if we use 'chunking' strategies to help us store and recall rhythmic patterns, this still makes us use our memory to a greater extent than we would generally do for processing speech.

Adaptability

According to Degé, one of the essential attributes of music-making is that it teaches people to be adaptive. To develop skills in making music or playing an instrument, a learner must constantly be in a state of learning and re-learning. For example, when first learning a rhythmic pattern or song, we might reproduce the timing or approximate 'shape' of a piece. This becomes the foundation, and as our brains form the new neural pathways, we then add detail – we might refine our timing or pitch; we might add dynamics; and as we become more adept, we might vary the tempo, improvise or transpose. Each iteration is 'correct' but different, and we may need to unlearn our earlier version to proceed. To make progress, we must update our concept of what is correct as we refine our skills.

This idea of needing to adapt highlights why we – as teachers, educators and facilitators – must regularly evaluate students' skills and help them progress to the next level. Using the OPERA hypothesis, we need to support precision but must carefully select the goal so that we do not risk losing attention, and engagement and, thereby, inhibit repetition. We need to be vigilant to signs of progress and be quick to reinforce and support small steps forwards. Degé highlights the need for feedback as part of adaptation – an issue that others have stressed as paramount in developing singing skills (e.g. Welch, 1985; Berglin, Pfordresher & Demorest, 2021).

Attention to temporal scales

Finally, the rhythm-specific PRISM theory (Fiveash *et al.*, 2021) highlights another set of skills and abilities needed to assist the transfer of rhythm skills to verbal learning. We must support attention to different 'layers' of rhythm – from rhythms that take place relatively slowly (such as metrical accent, phrases in language) to faster, more fine-grained levels (such as cues that mark syllables in speech or differentiate clusters of notes). (See Video 4 in the online resources for more about this.) As we learn to shift attention between layers, we adapt: we listen to the

MAKING MUSIC WORK FOR SPEECH AND WELLBEING

same piece of music in different ways and re-learn it. However, we need a sizeable auditory memory to hear rhythms that take place over a long period (see Chapters 2 and 3) such as metrical accent or the rhythmic pattern of a musical phrase. We must think about how we scaffold attention to layers of rhythm when working with young children, who have shorter auditory memories, or adult learners who have difficulties with auditory memory.

Section summary and implications

In conclusion, we must pay attention to each element of OPERA if we are to support musical development and expect new skills to transfer across domains, from music to speech. The most crucial – and challenging – condition is attention. Attention is key to developing precision and engaging the networks for music and speech. We can support attention when learning new skills by reducing task demands, by keeping training periods short and focused. We can stretch and challenge attention periodically, to support the executive function skills that most strongly benefit language. However, we must also be aware that some learners will face challenges in attention and sensory skills; these factors need specific consideration and may affect how easily or quickly learning transfers. We must also encourage adaptation in learning; teaching variations to songs or music will help learners re-learn, keeping activities fresh and engaging.

MUSIC, WELLBEING AND ACHIEVING 'FLOW'

Although we need to develop accuracy in musical skills, we must also support a learner's continuing enjoyment of music and help them reap the benefits of music as a tool for wellbeing. This means we must find a balance between challenge and achievability. The ideal learning state is one of 'flow' (Csikszentmihalyi, 1990), a condition in which we are focused and absorbed in an activity. Flow is a positive emotional state associated with happiness, relaxation and a sense of control. According to Csikszentmihalyi, people in this state use their skills 'to the utmost'. As such, flow is a desirable state to support the OPERA conditions. In flow, learners will apply their skills with engagement and light but focused attention. The state of flow is rewarding and will lead to repetition. To achieve a flow state, the task must be challenging enough to maintain focus and attention but not so tough that the task becomes stressful. As we monitor the learner's responses to tasks, we can reduce the challenge by going back to a less demanding activity, or providing additional sensory or cognitive support; or we can increase the task by moving to the next stage of development, shifting attention to a different level or layer, or by introducing tasks that require greater motor precision, vocal skill or memory. I will provide an example of how you can do this later in this section. Also see Appendices 1–4 and Video series 7 in the online resources.

Why make music with others?

Music-making is particularly well suited to supporting wellbeing when it involves other people (Koelsch, 2014; Croom, 2015). Many studies show emotional and social benefits for adults and children (e.g. Chadwick, 2010; Wood *et al.*, 2013; Perkins *et al.*, 2020). People who participate in group music activities feel connected with others and that they are working towards something bigger than themselves. Synchronizing movements with others, such as dancing, clapping, tapping or playing, is particularly pleasurable and can promote trust, compassion, empathy, cooperation and communication. Making music together can also lead to 'co-pathy', the sharing of emotions: that is, a change in mood in one member of the group may be 'caught' by another.

Specific activities may lend themselves easily to feelings of flow and wellbeing. Activities such as group drumming are especially beneficial for wellbeing, and can help learners get ready to learn. People who drum as part of a group describe how drumming can 'ground' them; they attribute the feelings of connection and calm that group drumming promotes to its simplicity and earthiness (Perkins *et al.*, 2016). Drumming also fosters feelings of social connection and offers non-verbal means of communication. For some, drumming can produce a state of flow that induces altered states of consciousness, akin to trance, meditation or spiritual experiences. Studies have shown that 15 minutes of repetitive drumming can lead to changes in brain waves found in meditation and sleep – the changes in brainwaves are associated with states of being calm, alert, and relaxed and being 'present' (Jovanov & Maxfield, 2011). In this way, drumming can prepare young people for learning; once a calm but alert state is achieved, drumming can become a tool to support rhythm skills for speech or practise advanced skills in inhibition, task-switching, dual-motor skills and focused attention (see Videos series 7 and Video 10 in the online resources for practical examples of using these skills).

Singing produces numerous benefits to wellbeing. The act of singing exercises the respiratory muscles, promoting optimal deep breathing patterns and improving heart rate variability. Endorphins are released, promoting a feeling of happiness. Regular singers report feelings of energy, joy, reduction in stress and improved concentration. Much of the research has focused on older adults, but a study with three-to five-year-old children from disadvantaged backgrounds showed lower cortisol measures – indicative of reduced stress – after weekly arts sessions involving music, dance and art, than a group of children who received within-class activities. As with drumming, adults and children perceive social and emotional benefits from group singing. Importantly for children with communication difficulties, this sense of collective belonging that occurs in group singing comes from taking part – that is, the benefits are not dependent on skill or output.

MUSIC, LANGUAGE AND CULTURAL CONNECTION

Furthermore, singing and drumming are universal. Through simple music-making, we can help the young people we work with to feel connected with others in their group, and with the wider global community. In Chapter 1, we began by tracing the history of music in healing and communication to ancient Greece; we could extend this story back into prehistory, too, as evidenced by archaeological records of musical instruments and vocal capacity (e.g. see Steven Mithen, *The Singing Neanderthals* (2005)). Through music, we can share stories and experiences, and connect across time, geographical distance, culture and religion. In this way, music makes us feel deeply connected with the human experience; this, too, offers benefits for wellbeing. In Chapter 3 we also looked at the importance of enculturation in developing musical skills, and how immersion in the music of other cultures is as valuable to our brains as a rich linguistic experience. Dr Hadiza Kere Abdulrahman, Lecturer and Founder of Fun House Prep School in Nigeria, gives us insight into these ideas, as she reflects on the role of music in her own culture.

Music, language and culture

REFLECTIONS ON THE PLACE OF MUSIC IN AFRICAN CULTURES

Dr Hadiza Kere Abdulrahman, Lecturer in Special Educational Needs, Disability and Inclusion, and Founder of Funhouse Prep School, Nigeria

In many African settings, the use of music and songs is ubiquitous and often starts very early in all activities and spheres. African children are exposed to songs very early on, from their times on their mothers' backs to the moments of watching their mothers undertake common household activities like pounding, grinding and washing. There is often a song for every activity. In the night times, there are special folktales and stories packed with songs filled with teachings, warnings, life and moral lessons. Nketia as far back as 1974 observed how the African mother sings to her child and introduces the child to music right from the cradle. Emeka (1994) later noted how African children generally improved their language and number skills by playing musical and rhythmic games while doing household chores or running errands.

The above highlights the deep-rooted place of music in African cultures, from homes to non-formal learning settings, and raises the question of the use of music generally as a pedagogical tool. The use of music for teaching can be found even in alternative schooling systems like the classical Qur'anic schools of Muslim West Africa. Arabic letters used for learning the Qur'an are domesticated into local languages and fashioned into sing-songs to make them into mnemonics; this, in turn, helps with recitation and memorization which are key pedagogical practices for this form of schooling. From my own personal reflections, I come from a very musical culture, the Nupe/Hausa people of northern Nigeria, and I have very early memories of folktales involving music, told by my mother and extended family members. I still remember the stories and songs many decades later, and the lessons contained within. My mother in turn, recalls rich stories handed down to her by her father and grandmother before her; she remembers times of singing and dancing under the moonlight when that was the only form of entertainment. Africa has a rich history of oral traditions – both spoken and sung – and in all of its cultures there are different songs for every occasion, from birth to death, through joys and sadness, and our lives are the richer for this.

Take the well-known African talking drum, for instance, also known as dundun in the Yoruba language of Nigeria. Analysis by Durojaye *et al.* (2021) into the acoustical similarities between the Yoruba language vocalizations and the talking drum found a high degree of correlation. The talking drum mimicked the microstructure of the tonal language. The study highlighted how this speech surrogacy served a number of functions, from disseminating oral history to reciting poetry and proverbs, adding that through musical instruments like these drums, one can learn the history of a particular culture as well as aspects of what people think, their belief systems, values and what is likely to be important to them. This supports the earlier assertion of the role of music in not only communication but also enculturation. The study also emphasized the value of studying non-Western cultures in order to understand various phenomena in mainstream musicology and linguistics that go beyond Western domains. Onyiuke (2005) had earlier called for a revisiting of African traditional paradigms to help in determining norms for effective childhood music education in particular. This is increasingly relevant for decolonizing music and music education in general.

In conclusion, my reflections reiterate the need to highlight and tease out common uses of music for learning and socialization generally. In many cultures, the educational and social uses of music are so commonplace that they risk being taken for granted as powerful tools for communication, education and enculturation. Active reflections about the value of music in our own culture help to connect some of those dots.

Hadiza's reflections eloquently capture so many ideas that we have explored in this book, such as the commonality of music, how we use music to connect with each other and teach, and how music – especially rhythm – can be a substitute for speech. Her words highlight how *holistic* music is, whereas I have deliberately and artificially broken music into parts. This fragmentation has helped us learn what each separate part of music can do for the different elements of language, and given us space to explore how we can adapt what we do to help young people master these separate, foundational skills. It is now time to put the pieces back together and think about how we can use music in a more spontaneous and fun way while remaining mindful of how we could tweak *this* element or *that* to support the learner's musical skills and improve the potential for skills to transfer to speech. In the sections below, I give examples of how you can use drumming and singing activities in these ways. I suggest you try the activities yourself so you understand how you are using your different cognitive, attentional and emotional skills. Appendices 2–4 in the online resources contain additional examples and sample programmes of music, tailored to different levels of musical and verbal ability.

HOW DO WE MAKE MUSICAL LEARNING 'JUST RIGHT' FOR TRANSFER AND WELLBEING?

The example below shows how we might use a drumming activity to enable all aspects of the OPERA and PRISM hypotheses. The activity requires attention and precision, and awareness of pulse, rhythm, meter and timbre. To someone who enjoys drumming, the activity is emotionally rewarding. It can also encourage a calm, meditative state, support verbal learning, and prime the speech centres for speech.

TRY THIS YOURSELF

In the sequence of videos When the Rain Comes (Video series 7), I provide examples of the activity using household objects – you could use these to try this yourself, at different levels of complexity, by working through the steps below. As you do play, think about how you would adapt the activity for the young person or people you work with.

Drumming to support verbal learning and wellbeing: example.

Let us imagine a neurotypical, able-bodied child or adult as they play a word-based rhythm with another learner and achieve a sense of flow.

The young person is drumming a complex sequence of hand movements based on a verbal phrase (example: *when the rain comes, when the rain comes down*). They *alternate left- and right-hand movements*, beginning with their dominant hand; at the same time, they shift their hands, so *they make some sounds in the centre of the drum and some close to the rim of the drum*; they regulate the pressure of their taps to *vary the intensity of the sound*. To begin with, they *mentally rehearse the words* as they drum, playing slowly as they master the movement patterns and motor coordination. When they have started to develop motor-memory, they need not concentrate so hard on mentally repeating the words and can *begin to play at a faster tempo*.

Now, we introduce another element to increase the challenge: they must maintain their rhythm but *play against a second rhythm* (such as 'where is my umbrella?'). To do this – and to maintain flow – they need to keep a 'light' concentration on their own rhythm and on the second pattern. Their attention must be on what they are doing while remaining aware of their sound against another. However, if they overthink their movements or worry about doing them right, their thoughts will intrude into their phonological loop (see Chapter 2), upsetting their mental rehearsal and the coordination of their hands. The flow state comes when the rhythm is just challenging enough that they must keep focused, but not so challenging that they become stressed or have too many demands on their working memory or cognitive processing.

When the Goldilocks moment is in place, we can introduce a new challenge – add in another factor to increase their attention, memory and focus, or direct their attention to a different layer of rhythm. For example, we might ask them to *alternate patterns* by playing a previously well-rehearsed pattern and the newly learned pattern; *tap to the strong beat* with their foot as they play; *accent the strong beats* with greater clarity; or *lead with the non-dominant hand*. These types of activities make their brains work hard. They must use their auditory memory, motor coordination and motor timing, and they must remain focused while ignoring competing information (attentional inhibition). When they reach the Goldilocks moment and can keep playing in a lightly focused state, they feel engaged and rewarded; they may also experience positive emotions. This state is ideal for supporting the transfer of learning across domains, as it motivates them to repeat the activity, fulfilling each criterion of OPERA (Patel, 2011, 2014).

Adapting rhythm tasks

A learner with physical or sensory differences might face more challenges than the adult I describe above. However, we can do a lot to make the tasks manageable while always working to develop their skills in attention, focus, and motor timing. We can adjust the demands of a task by directing the child's focus to specific aspects of their activity. For example, to simplify the task and reduce the amount of sensory information they must process, we could play the same rhythm with them, or say or sing the words as they play. We might gradually quieten and stop, let them continue unsupported for as long as they can, and then come back to play with them. To increase demands, we might ask them to play against the pulse; or we might ask them to walk the pulse as they say or play the rhythm. As we saw in Chapter 4, our motor abilities tend to deteriorate when we need to split our attention, but being able to perform multiple activities (e.g. move and sing) is a valuable skill for music, and it encourages the brain to work hard.

Let us look at some of the ways we can adapt this task to simplify it, and help a learner develop skills gradually. The example below shows how you might teach the activity in small steps:

Step 1: Focus on posture and proprioception. Ideally, we need to be in a good posture for playing and singing (see Chapter 6). However, for some learners, postural control can be a demanding task. They may not be able to pay attention to posture and performance without losing control over one or both domains. It is important to consider how and when to support attention to posture. For example, encourage posture awareness while playing along to a simple beat or rhythm. Do not focus on the accuracy of the learner's motor timing at this stage, but encourage them to become aware of their 'best' body posture and arm movement while playing (this could follow on from Tracey's exercises to support stability, in Chapter 6; see Videos 8 and 9 in the online resources). If necessary, guide the learner into the ideal postural position and support them there as they play to encourage the feel of good posture. Encourage independence but build postural awareness and control gradually.

Step 2: Focus on motor timing accuracy. Next, shift attention to accuracy in motor timing. Maybe let the learner change position to relieve postural muscles, or use stability aids (splints, or compression clothing) so the body is supported as much as possible. Now direct the learner to focus on the accuracy of their timing – give them feedback on how they are doing, but encourage them to use feedback from their own body; ask them to close their eyes and listen to their own rhythm against the target beat; ask them to feel the movement of their hands on the drum – can they make the taps more precise, quieter, louder? The aim here is to encourage sensory and auditory awareness while minimizing additional – unnecessary – sensory information and processing. You can try a slower or faster tempo and see how motor timing is affected. Is there an optimum tempo? If so, work at the learner's best tempo to encourage accuracy, then adjust the tempo – a slower tempo is more demanding in terms of cognition (e.g. memory, self-regulation) and motor control, whereas a faster tempo will be more challenging for motor coordination. Through varying this, you can keep challenging different skills for learning.

Step 3: Introduce words. Now we can begin to engage auditory-verbal memory and prime the brain for speech. Teach a new rhythm, based on words – this can be chosen by you or the learner, or selected from any music resource. You might be able to use rhythmic patterns and phrases that exceed the learner's auditory memory capacity because rhythm helps us 'chunk' verbal information, and an audible beat and rhythm can assist both attention and memory for rhythm. However, if you know the auditory digit span of the learner, work to this: make the word or phrase suitable for their digit span, but do not make it so long that it causes them to feel anxious or stressed. For example, if a child or adult has a digit span of four, try a rhythm that is based on four words, or a phrase with five or six syllables that can be 'chunked' over four beats in a bar (see Figure 10.1). Ideally, you want to use phrases that capture the natural rhythms of speech. The example we used earlier ('When the Rain Comes') fits into four beats and captures the durational pattern of conversation, but it has complex timing. A phrase like *I feel happy now* (whose rhythm is *ta ta tee-tee ta*) is simpler, and begins on a strong beat. Have fun creating your own word-based rhythms and seeing how they fit together.

TIMING AND MEMORY IN 'WHEN THE RAIN COMES DOWN'

The rhythm *when the rain comes down* has five syllables that fit into a bar of four beats (Figure 10.1). As such, most children and young people should be able to perceive the phrase if their auditory memory is close to 4 digits. However, the rhythm poses challenges for beginners, as the words 'when the' come before the strong beat, an example of anacrusis: a technique of placing unstressed rhythms in music and poetry ahead of the stressed sound – see Figure 10.1. Additionally, the duration of 'rain' is longer in phrase one than phrase two: this activity is useful to help learners focus on perceiving and producing the types of subtle durational change that occurs in language (see Chapter 3), but performing the subtle changes can be challenging. You could perform this as call-and-response: you play phrase one, and the learner responds with phrase 2.

1	2	3	4
			(sh) *When the* Ti-ri ♫
rain Too-oo 𝅗𝅥		comes Ta ♩	(sh) *When the* Ti-ri ♫
rain Ta ♩	comes Ta ♩	down Ta ♩	

Figure 10.1: 'When the Rain Comes Down'. The figure shows how the words fit to a four-beat meter. The words 'when the' come on the final beat of the song, just before the strong beat (Beat 1, marked in bold type). The figure shows the rhythm syllables and standard notation for the rhythm in 4/4 time.

Step 4: Introduce the voice. Next, introduce the intonational melody of the word-phrase – hum it or use a neutral vowel/syllable as you play the rhythm; encourage the learner to do this, too, but again, see how this affects their motor timing. If they can simultaneously tap the rhythm and hum, ask them to use the words. Even for a neurotypical, able-bodied adult, this is challenging, so be prepared to simplify or go back a stage. Our aim is to maintain precision in that Goldilocks state.

Alternative approach: Start with the words. Some learners might find it easier to begin with the words by speaking them aloud, and then learning to internalize the patterns. For some learners, you might build these skills gradually, for example:

1. Prime the words by clapping their rhythm.
2. Say the words and clap their rhythm.
3. Ask the student to repeat the words verbally.
4. Ask them to say the words as you provide an audible beat (support word recall with visuals if needed).
5. Ask them to say and clap the words.
6. Ask them to 'whisper the words' and clap them.
7. Ask them to 'think' the words and clap them.
8. Progress to playing word rhythms.

(NOTE: This process might take a few sessions, depending on the learner.)

How might I use a singing activity to develop skills for speech?

A similar process can be used for singing activities. Until postural awareness and stability are built up, it may be difficult to sing while maintaining good posture, so focus on one or the other until the learner can integrate both skills. When first attempting singing with postural awareness, you may need to simplify the oro-motor movements – go back to humming, kazooing or vocalizing until posture and rhythm are consolidated. Alternatively, allow the learner to drop attention to one element (e.g. posture) to allow focus on word rhythm and voice. When singing, be ready to support attention, focus and memory with prompts (gesture, Makaton, written word) as skills are developing; and support posture as necessary – lying down while singing is acceptable and can offer benefits by relieving physical stress and increasing somatosensory feedback (see Chapter 7). An example is given in the online resources that shows how a singing game can be used for multiple purposes, and below (Table 10.1) I suggest ways to teach a song in discrete steps that link explicitly to transfer skills.

Table 10.1: Using a song to teach skills that can support verbal development and transfer to speech

Skills for transfer	Musical goal	Speech-related goal	Steps	Adaptations
Develop awareness of rhythm at different hierarchies	Play with metrical awareness	Attend to changes in rhythm at phrase level	Move with another to strongly metrical music – 2/2/, 3/4/, 4/4/, 6/8	Be rocked/bounced/swung
Involve physical movement for sensory integration and embodiment		Find ways to embody and show the strong beat – stamp it, shout it, clap it	Find ways to embody and show the strong beat – stamp it, shout it, clap it	
Practise 'adaptation' as part of developing executive function		Walk to a pulse and emphasize the strong beat – bigger movement, louder sound	Walk to a pulse and emphasize the strong beat – bigger movement, louder sound	Support physical and sensory needs as necessary – e.g. use coloured scarves and movements over volume
		Play to a pulse and show the strong beat	Play to a pulse and show the strong beat	Use visuals to show the stronger beat (e.g. a 'thicker' heart)
		Learner listens to you play a pulse and they must show the strong beat	Learner listens to you play a pulse and they must show the strong beat	Bounce a ball on the strong beat; feel a stronger pull on a large scrunchie; make a bigger wave in a scarf
		Learner conducts a metrical pulse at fast/slow tempi	Learner conducts a metrical pulse at fast/slow tempi	

Develop awareness of rhythm at different hierarchies	Reproduce rhythmic changes in song	Attend to rhythmic changes in language at phrase and syllable levels	Show an isochronous pulse and tap along to a song	
Involve physical movement for sensory integration and embodiment			Tap along to the pulse and listen to the melodic/rhythmic shape of the song (emphasize the big picture rather than discrete syllabic rhythms)	
Practise 'adaptation' as part of developing executive function			Listen to and watch the melodic shape (one neutral syllable, or an 'oo')	Provide visual shape of the melody in any form that works; consider a tactile representation – draw the shape on a hand
			Listen to and 'draw' the melodic shape (one neutral syllable)	Use objects (e.g. toys, puppets), gestures, pens; consider assisted movement, or whole-body movement
			Learner imitates the melodic shape	Consider using kazoos, humming, vowel sounds

cont.

Skills for transfer	Musical goal	Speech-related goal	Steps	Adaptations
Attention shifts to syllabic level	Play rhythm of words	Prime words and syllables for speech	Learner listens to and sees the rhythm emphasized within the melodic shape – consider singing the vowels of words without the consonants	Graphic scores (long/short lines)
			Learner imitates the rhythmic pattern of a phrase	Continue with graphic scores
			Teach the words: clap the pattern then sing the words in the phrase	
			Sing the song together	Tap the pulse gently/play a game – encourage internalization of words
			Learner plays with you as you all play the rhythm pattern and sing	
			Teach rhythm notation	
			Sing and play/clap the words together	Perform from graphic score/notation; support memory with images/actions/prompts

Begin to divide attention	Produce two 'levels' of rhythm		Learner plays the rhythm pattern as you play a pulse	Support memory as necessary
		Practise dual motor skills	Learner sings the song to a steady beat	Support memory as necessary
			Learner sings the song and moves to a steady beat	Learner might walk, clap, nod, tap or conduct
Encourage internalization of rhythm	Practise oro-motor skills for speech		Learner sings and plays the rhythm	Support auditory-verbal memory as necessary
			Learner sings solo – internal beat	Support auditory-verbal memory as necessary – then gradually reduce prompts
Practise transfer			Learner speaks the words	Provide an external beat or rhythm to support, if necessary

STRUCTURING A SESSION TO BALANCE
LEARNING WITH WELLBEING

For people who have significant language delays and differences, music lessons should be intensive (e.g. see Swaminathan & Schellenberg, 2020) for learning to transfer between domains. This means practice should be regular and focused. However, we need to keep intensive practice periods short, especially if we are working with learners who are still developing the ability to sustain attention. We must alternate intense concentration with rest to reduce the negative effects of cognitive load. A practical way to do this is to switch activities regularly. Avoid repeating a similar activity within the same session, too: our brains can become confused if we try to improve more than one motor skill at a time, impeding learning (Sousa, 2016). Table 10.2 shows how you might structure activities to create this rhythm between focused and light work. Some of the books, below, offer programmes that you can adapt, and I include example programmes with suggested adaptations in Appendices 1–4 – you may download, print and use them as you like.

Table 10.2: Example of how to structure a session to alternate focused learning with relaxed learning

Activity	Purposes
Relaxed activity: warm up the body – e.g. dance to music	Energize, feel the beat, enjoy
Focused practice: posture for breath and voice; breathwork	Develop muscle groups needed for movement and voice
Relaxed practice: kazoo along to a pop song, draw shapes of the melody in the air, mime the words using big mouth shapes, play air guitars to a beat or rhythm	Have fun, listen to and show the beat, rhythms and melodic shape of a familiar song; move the articulators
Focused practice: vocal exercises e.g. sustained vowels using SOVT, pitch glides, scales	Develop skills in 'easy' phonation, use and strengthen the vocal muscles
Relaxed practice: play a singing game, e.g. action song or game	Become familiar with a new song while having fun
Focused practice: listen to the new song and tap or move to the beat	Show beat timing and entrainment skills while listening and learning

CONCLUSIONS

We began the book by considering whether music can support the language skills of learners with developmental or sensory differences, or even if learners with complex needs can become better musicians. I hope I have shown you that there is much potential for using music for verbal skills, and more. Some learners will face ongoing difficulties with language and speech – and music – that will slow or alter musical development. Music will not banish these, or transform skills: for our learners – as much as for professional musicians – transfer depends on skill development, and skill development requires focused periods of attention, and lots of practice.

As parents, teachers and facilitators, we can help children and young people to develop their musical skills by encouraging precision and focus, and by adapting our teaching and support to reduce the effects of some of the barriers they face. Typically, we might need to change the pace of our delivery, reduce or increase the types of sensory feedback (like turning up or down the signals to their body), and provide ways to challenge certain skills, while managing or minimizing excessive cognitive demands (depending on our learning aim). We must be patient: some changes might appear very quickly but others could take years. We need to be open to different ways of hearing and sensing music; we need to become good observers, and excellent at giving feedback; we need to be willing to do everything ourselves and challenge ourselves as much as we challenge our learners; and we need to imbue it all with a sense of playfulness and fun, especially when doing the serious work.

You probably picked up this book knowing just how powerful music is for the learners you work with. I hope that the science and research in this book have helped you understand *why* music offers so much to all of us, and that I have highlighted its potential for developing verbal skills, and shown you how you can adapt music-making activities to meet different learning needs. However, research often lags behind practice, especially for learners with complex needs. The next stage of this story lies with you – try some of the ideas in this book and test them; use whatever music books and instruments you have to hand, adapting them as needed. Be excited at what music can offer, but sceptical as to whether it will make a difference. Look out for every sign of success or failure; especially failure, as that forces us to rethink and adapt, and to carry on learning about our learners.

Thank you for joining me on my journey, and good luck to you and your learners as you make music for verbal learning. I would love to hear how you get on!

RECOMMENDED READING
Music activities

Bean, J. & Oldfield, A. (2001). *Pied Piper: Musical Activities to Develop Basic Skills*. London: Jessica Kingsley Publishers.

Corke, M. (2014). *Approaches to Communication through Music*. London: Routledge.

Houlahan, M. & Tacka, P. (2015). *Kodály Today: A Cognitive Approach to Elementary Music Education*. Oxford: Oxford University Press.

Ockelford, A. (2008). *Music for Children and Young People with Complex Needs*. Oxford: Oxford University Press.

Ott, P. (2011). *Music for Special Kids: Musical Activities, Songs, Instruments and Resources*. London: Jessica Kingsley Publishers.

Ramey, M. (2011). *Group Music Activities for Adults with Intellectual and Developmental Disabilities*. London: Jessica Kingsley Publishers.

Stormont, B. & Shepard, C. (2004). *Jabulani!: Ideas for Making Music (Education Series)*. Stroud: Hawthorn Press.

Music, wellbeing, communication

Cudd, S. (2020). The Perceived Benefits of Participation in Community Drum Circles. Masters' thesis, Catherine University, St Paul, Minnesota.

Williamson, V. (2014). *You Are the Music: How Music Reveals What It Means to Be Human*. London: Icon Books.

MacDonald, R., Kreutz, G. & Mitchell, L. (eds) (2013). *Music, Health, and Wellbeing*. Oxford: Oxford University Press.

Bibliography

Ab Shukor, N.F., Han, W., Lee, J. & Seo, Y.J. (2021). Crucial music components needed for speech perception enhancement of pediatric cochlear implant users: A systematic review and meta-analysis. *Audiology and Neurotology*, 1–25.

Abdoola, S., Botha, A., Van der Linde, J. & Ras, E. (2017). Dysphonia in adults with developmental stuttering: A descriptive study. *South African Journal of Communication Disorders*, 64(1), 1–7.

Aichert, I., Lehner, K., Falk, S., Späth, M. & Ziegler, W. (2019). Do patients with neurogenic speech sound impairments benefit from auditory priming with a regular metrical pattern? *Journal of Speech, Language, and Hearing Research*, 62(8S), 3104–3118.

Aitchison, J. (2012). *Words in the Mind: An Introduction to the Mental Lexicon*. Hoboken, NJ: John Wiley & Sons.

Albarrati, A.M., Alghamdi, M.S.M., Nazer, R.I., Alkorashy, M.M., Alshowier, N. & Gale, N. (2018). Effectiveness of low to moderate physical exercise training on the level of low-density lipoproteins: A systematic review. *BioMed Research International*, 2018, 5982980.

Albertini, G., Bonassi, S., Dall'Armi, V., Giachetti, I., Giaquinto, S. & Mignano, M. (2010). Spectral analysis of the voice in Down syndrome. *Research in Developmental Disabilities*, 31(5), 995–1001.

Alexandrou, A.M., Saarinen, T., Kujala, J. & Salmelin, R. (2016). A multimodal spectral approach to characterize rhythm in natural speech. *The Journal of the Acoustical Society of America*, 139(1), 215–226.

Alm, P.A. (2004). Stuttering and the basal ganglia circuits: A critical review of possible relations. *Journal of Communication Disorders*, 37(4), 325–369. http://doi.org/10.1016/j.jcomdis.2004.03.001.

Alves-Pinto, A., Turova, V., Blumenstein, T. & Lampe, R. (2016). The case for musical instrument training in cerebral palsy for neurorehabilitation. *Neural Plasticity*, 2016: 1072301. doi: 10.1155/2016/1072301.

Amos, P. (2013). Rhythm and timing in autism: Learning to dance. *Frontiers in Integrative Neuroscience*, 7, 27.

Aronson, A.E. & Bless, D.M. (2009). *Clinical Voice Disorders*. New York. NY: Thieme.

Arulanandam, S., Hakim, A.J., Aziz, Q., Sandhu, G. & Birchall, M.A. (2017). Laryngological presentations of Ehlers-Danlos syndrome: Case series of nine patients from two London tertiary referral centres. *Clinical Otolaryngology*, 42(4), 860–863.

Assaneo, M.F. & Poeppel, D. (2018). The coupling between auditory and motor cortices is rate-restricted: Evidence for an intrinsic speech-motor rhythm. *Science Advances*, 4(2), eaao3842.

Aubanel, V., Davis, C. & Kim, J. (2016). Exploring the role of brain oscillations in speech perception in noise: intelligibility of isochronously retimed speech. *Frontiers in Human Neuroscience*, 10, 430.

Ayres, J.G., Pope, F.M., Reidy, J.F. & Clark, T.J.H. (1985). Abnormalities of the lungs and thoracic cage in the Ehlers-Danlos syndrome. *Thorax*, 40(4), 300–305. https://doi.org/10.1136/thx.40.4.300.

Azekawa, M. & Lagasse, A.B. (2018). Singing exercises for speech and vocal abilities in individuals with hypokinetic dysarthria: A feasibility study. *Music Therapy Perspectives*, 36(1), 40–49.

Barkley, R.A. (2011). The important role of executive functioning and self-regulation in ADHD. *Journal of Child Neuropsychology*, 113(21), 41–56.

Barkley, R.A. (2022). Improving clinical diagnosis using the executive functioning: Self-regulation theory of ADHD. *The ADHD Report*, 30(1), 1–9.

Barks, L. & Shaw, P. (2011). Wheelchair positioning and breathing in children with cerebral palsy: Study methods and lessons learned. *Rehabilitation Nursing*, 36(4), 146–152.

Barona-Lleo, L. & Fernandez, S. (2016). Hyperfunctional voice disorder in children with Attention Deficit Hyperactivity Disorder (ADHD). A phenotypic characteristic? *Journal of Voice*, 30(1), 114–119.

Baron-Cohen, S., Johnson, D., Asher, J., Wheelwright, S. *et al.* (2013). Is synaesthesia more common in autism? *Molecular Autism*, 4(1), 1–6.

Bateson, M.C. (1975). Mother-infant exchanges: the epigenesis of conversational interaction. *Annals of the New York Academy of Sciences*, 263(1), 101–113.

Bean, J. & Oldfield, A. (2001). *Pied Piper: Musical Activities to Develop Basic Skills*. London: Jessica Kingsley Publishers.

Beaumont, D., Blakely, T., Stuart, N. & Woodward, J. (2021). Increasing engagement for young children with autism spectrum disorder using Way to Play: A preliminary investigation of the adult training program. *Australasian Journal of Special and Inclusive Education*, 1–13. https://doi.org/10.1017/jsi.2021.14.

Beck, K. (2010). Organic Variation of the Vocal Apparatus. In Hardcastle, W.J., Laver, J. and Gibbon, F.E. (eds), *The Handbook of Phonetic Sciences* (second edition), pp.155–201. Hoboken, NJ: Wiley-Blackwell.

Berger, D.S. (2002). *Music Therapy, Sensory Integration and the Autistic Child*. London: Jessica Kingsley Publishers.

Berger, D.S. (2015). *Eurhythmics for Autism and Other Neurophysiologic Diagnoses: A Sensorimotor Music-Based Treatment Approach*. London: Jessica Kingsley Publishers.

Bergeson, T.R. & Trehub, S.E. (2006). Infants' perception of rhythmic patterns. *Music Perception*, 23(4), 345–360.

Berglin, J., Pfordresher, P.Q. & Demorest, S. (2021). The effect of visual and auditory feedback on adult poor-pitch remediation. *Psychology of Music*, 50(4), 1077–1090.

Bertrand, P., Navarro, H., Caussade, S., Holmgren, N. & Sánchez, I. (2003). Airway anomalies in children with Down syndrome: Endoscopic findings. *Pediatric Pulmonology*, 36(2), 137–141.

Besson, M., Chobert, J. & Marie, C. (2011). Transfer of training between music and speech: Common processing, attention, and memory. *Frontiers in Psychology*, 2(May), 94. http://doi.org/10.3389/ fpsyg.2011.00094.

Bharathi, G., Jayaramayya, K., Balasubramanian, V. & Vellingiri, B. (2019). The potential role of rhythmic entrainment and music therapy intervention for individuals with autism spectrum disorders. *Journal of Exercise Rehabilitation*, 15(2), 180.

Bispham, J. (2006). Rhythm in music: What is it? Who has it? And why? *Music Perception*, 24(2), 125–134.

Blain-Moraes, S., Chesser, S., Kingsnorth, S., McKeever, P. & Biddiss, E. (2013). Biomusic: A novel technology for revealing the personhood of people with profound multiple disabilities. *Augmentative and Alternative Communication*, 29(2), 159–173.

Blasi, A., Lloyd-Fox, S., Sethna, V., Brammer, M.J. *et al.* (2015). Atypical processing of voice sounds in infants at risk for autism spectrum disorder. *Cortex*, 71, 122–133.

Boada, R., Willcutt, E.G. & Pennington, B.F. (2012). Understanding the comorbidity between dyslexia and attention-deficit/hyperactivity disorder. *Topics in Language Disorders*, 32(3), 264–284.

Boel, L., Pernet, K., Toussaint, M., Ides, K. *et al.* (2019). Respiratory morbidity in children with cerebral palsy: An overview. *Developmental Medicine & Child Neurology*, 61(6), 646–653.

Borrie, S.A., Lubold, N. & Pon-Barry, H. (2015). Disordered speech disrupts conversational entrainment: A study of acoustic-prosodic entrainment and communicative success in populations with communication challenges. *Frontiers in Psychology*, 6, 1187.

Boyce-Tillman, J. (2000). *Constructing Musical Healing: The Wounds that Sing*. London: Jessica Kingsley Publishers.

Bravi, R., Cohen, E.J., Martinelli, A., Gottard, A. & Minciacchi, D. (2017). When non-dominant is better than dominant: Kinesiotape modulates asymmetries in timed performance during a synchronization-continuation task. *Frontiers in Integrative Neuroscience*, 11, 21.

Bresee, C. (2019). Examining Music as a Tool for Facilitating the Use of Augmentative and Alternative Communication for Students with Multiple Disabilities Including Extensive Intellectual Disabilities, Orthopedic Impairments, and Visual Impairments: A Case Story. Masters' thesis, California State University, St Marcos.

Bricout, V.A., Pace, M., Dumortier, L., Favre-Juvin, A. & Guinot, M. (2018). Autonomic responses to head-up tilt test in children with autism spectrum disorders. *Journal of Abnormal Child Psychology*, 46(5), 1121–1128.

Bright, W. (1963). Language and music: Areas for cooperation. *Ethnomusicology*, 7(1), 26–32.

Broesch, T.L. & Bryant, G.A. (2015). Prosody in infant-directed speech is similar across western and traditional cultures. *Journal of Cognition and Development*, 16(1), 31–43.

Brooks, L.J., Olsen, M.N., Bacevice, A.M., Beebe, A., Konstantinopoulou, S. & Taylor, H.G. (2015). Relationship between sleep, sleep apnea, and neuropsychological function in children with Down syndrome. *Sleep and Breathing*, 19(1), 197–204.

Caçador, M. & Paço, J. (2018). The influence of posture and balance on voice: A review. *Gazeta Médica*, 2(5).

Caldwell, P. (2006). *Finding You Finding Me*. London: Jessica Kingsley Publishers.

Cason, N., Astésano, C. & Schön, D. (2015). Bridging music and speech rhythm: Rhythmic priming and audio–motor training affect speech perception. *Acta Psychologica*, 155, 43–50.

Cason, N., Hidalgo, C., Isoard, F., Roman, S. & Schön, D. (2015). Rhythmic priming enhances speech production abilities: Evidence from prelingually deaf children. *Neuropsychology*, 29(1), 102.

Castori, M. (2012). Ehlers-Danlos syndrome, hypermobility type: An underdiagnosed hereditary connective tissue disorder with mucocutaneous, articular, and systemic manifestations. *ISRN Dermatology*, 2012, 1–22. https://doi.org/10.5402/2012/751768.

Castori, M., Camerota, F., Celletti, C., Danese, C. *et al.* (2010). Natural history and manifestations of the hypermobility type Ehlers-Danlos syndrome: A pilot study on 21 patients. *American Journal of Medical Genetics*, 152(3), 556–564.

Celletti, C., Mari, G., Ghibellini, G., Celli, M., Castori, M. & Camerota, F. (2015). Phenotypic variability in developmental coordination disorder: Clustering of generalized joint hypermobility with attention deficit/hyperactivity disorder, atypical swallowing and narrative difficulties. *American Journal of Medical Genetics, Part C: Seminars in Medical Genetics,* 169(1), 117–122. https://doi.org/10.1002/ajmg.c.31427.

Chacona, S.M. (2008). Effect of world music drumming on auditory and visual attention skills of ADHD elementary students. *Dissertation Abstracts International: Section A: Humanities and Social Sciences*, 2008(68), 2817.

Chadwick, H.B. (2010). A rhythm for life: Drumming for wellbeing. *British Journal of Wellbeing*, 1(9), 13–15.

Chatzoudis, D., Kelly, T.J., Lancaster, J. & Jones, T.M. (2015). Upper airway obstruction in a patient with Ehlers-Danlos syndrome. *The Annals of The Royal College of Surgeons of England*, 97(3), e50–e51.

Cheung, S., Han, E., Kushki, A., Anagnostou, E. & Biddiss, E. (2016). Biomusic: An auditory interface for detecting physiological indicators of anxiety in children. *Frontiers in Neuroscience*, 10, 401.

Chen, J.C. (2016). *Elements of Human Voice*. Singapore: World Scientific.

Chu, S.Y. & Barlow, S.M. (2016). A call for biomechanics to understand hypotonia and speech movement disorders in Down syndrome. *Advances in Communication Disorder*, 16(1), 2–40.

Clark, A., Anderson, S., Hittner, E. & Kraus, N. (2012). Musical experience strengthens the neural representation of sounds important for communication in middle-aged adults. *Frontiers in Aging Neuroscience*, 4, 30.

Colling, L.J., Noble, H.L. & Goswami, U. (2017). Neural entrainment and sensorimotor synchronization to the beat in children with developmental dyslexia: An EEG study. *Frontiers in Neuroscience*, 11, 360.

Cope, T.E., Shtyrov, Y., MacGregor, L.J., Holland, R. *et al.* (2020). Anterior temporal lobe is necessary for efficient lateralised processing of spoken word identity. *Cortex*, 126, 107–118.

Corke, M. (2014). *Approaches to Communication through Music*. London: Routledge.

Cowell, P.E. (2010). Auditory Laterality: Recent Findings in Speech Perception. In K. Hugdahl & R. Westerhausen (eds), *The Two Halves of The Brain: Information Processing in the Cerebral Hemispheres*, pp.349–377. Cambridge, MA: MIT Press.

Croom, A.M. (2015). Music practice and participation for psychological well-being: A review of how music influences positive emotion, engagement, relationships, meaning, and accomplishment. *Musicae Scientiae*, 19(1), 44–64.

Csikszentmihalyi, M. (1990). *Flow: The Psychology of Optimal Experience*. New York, NY: Harper and Row.

Cudd, S. (2020). The Perceived Benefits of Participation in Community Drum Circles. Masters' thesis, Catherine University, St Paul, Minnesota.

Cumming, R.E. (2010). Speech Rhythm: The Language-Specific Integration of Pitch and Duration. Doctoral dissertation, University of Cambridge.

Cumming, R., Wilson, A., Leong, V., Colling, L.J. & Goswami, U. (2015). Awareness of rhythm patterns in speech and music in children with specific language impairments. *Frontiers in Human Neuroscience*, 9, 672.

Cummins, F. (2015). Rhythm and Speech. In M.A. Redford (ed.), *The Handbook of Speech Production*, pp.158–177. Chichester: John Wiley & Sons.

Degé, F. (2021). Music lessons and cognitive abilities in children: How far transfer could be possible. *Frontiers in Psychology*, 11, 3656.

Deutsch, D. (2003). Track 22. *On Phantom Words, and Other Curiosities* [CD]. La Jolla, CA: Philomel Records.

Deutsch, D. (2010). Speaking in tones. *Scientific American Mind*, 21(3), 36–43.

Dienerowitz, T., Peschel, T., Vogel, M., Poulain, T. *et al.* (2021). Establishing normative data on singing voice parameters of children and adolescents with average singing activity using the voice range profile. *Folia Phoniatrica et Logopaedica*, 1–12.

Dimon, T. (2018). *Anatomy of the Voice: An Illustrated Guide for Singers, Vocal Coaches, and Speech Therapists*. Berkeley, CA: North Atlantic Books.

Drake, C. & Gérard, C. (1989). A psychological pulse train: How young children use this cognitive framework to structure simple rhythms. *Psychological Research*, 51(1), 16–22.

Drake, C., Jones, M.R. & Baruch, C. (2000). The development of rhythmic attending in auditory sequences: Attunement, referent period, focal attending. *Cognition*, 77(3), 251–288.

Dumortier, L. & Bricout, V.A. (2020). Obstructive sleep apnea syndrome in adults with Down syndrome: Causes and consequences. Is it a 'chicken and egg' question? *Neuroscience & Biobehavioral Reviews*, 108, 124–138.

Durojaye, C., Knowles, K.L., Patten, K.J., Garcia, M.J. & McBeath, M.K. (2021). When music speaks: An acoustic study of the speech surrogacy of the Nigerian dùndún talking drum. *Frontiers in Communication*, https://doi.org/10.3389/fcomm.2021.652690.

Dworsky, A. (2013). *Slap Happy: How to Play World-Beat Rhythms with Just Your Body and a Buddy*. Santa Ynez, CA: Dancing Hands Music.

Eidsheim, N.S. (2015). *Sensing Sound*. Durham, NC: Duke University Press.

Ekins, C., Wright, J., Schulz, H., Wright, P.R., Owens, D. & Millder, W. (2019). Effects of a drums alive® kids beats intervention on motor skills and behavior in children with intellectual disabilities. *Palaestra*, 33(2).

Emeka, A.L.N. (1994). Culture Contact, Social Change, Ethnicity and Integration. In R.C. Okafor, L.N. Emeka & E. Akumah (eds), *Nigerian Peoples and Culture*, pp.104–123. Enugu: ESUTH.

Falk, S., Müller, T. & Dalla Bella, S. (2014). Sensorimotor synchronization in stuttering children and adolescents. *Procedia-Social and Behavioral Sciences*, 126, 206–207.

Faulkner, S. (2016). *Rhythm to Recovery: A Practical Guide to Using Rhythmic Music, Voice and Movement for Social and Emotional Development*. London: Jessica Kingsley Publishers.

Fedorowski, A. (2018). Postural orthostatic tachycardia syndrome: Clinical presentation, aetiology and management. *Journal of Internal Medicine*, 285(4), 352–366. https://doi.org/10.1111/joim.12852.

Ferguson, C.A. & Farwell, C.B. (1975). Words and sounds in early language acquisition. *Language*, 51(2), 419–439.

Fernando, T. & Goldman, R.D. (2019). Management of gastroesophageal reflux disease in pediatric patients with cerebral palsy. *Canadian Family Physician*, 65(11), 796–798.

Fisher, J. & Keyes, G. (2018). *This Is a Voice: 99 Exercises to Train, Project, and Harness the Power of Your Voice*. London: Wellcome Collection.

Fiveash, A., Bedoin, N., Gordon, R.L. & Tillmann, B. (2021). Processing rhythm in speech and music: Shared mechanisms and implications for developmental speech and language disorders. *Neuropsychology*, 35(8), 771.

Flaugnacco, E., Lopez, L., Terribili, C., Montico, M., Zoia, S. & Schön, D. (2015). Music training increases phonological awareness and reading skills in developmental dyslexia: A randomized control trial. *PloS One*, 10(9), e0138715.

Fotiadou, E., Giagazoglou, P., Kokaridas, D., Angelopoulou, N., Tsimaras, V. & Tsorbatzoudis, C. (2002). Effect of rhythmic gymnastics on the dynamic balance of children with deafness. *European Journal of Special Needs Education*, 17(3), 301–309.

Fotiadou, E.G., Neofotistou, K.H., Sidiropoulou, M.P., Tsimaras, V.K., Mandroukas, A.K. & Angelopoulou, N.A. (2009). The effect of a rhythmic gymnastics program on the dynamic balance ability of individuals with intellectual disability. *The Journal of Strength & Conditioning Research*, 23(7), 2102–2106.

Franco, F., Suttora, C., Spinelli, M., Kozar, I. & Fasolo, M. (2020). Singing to infants matters: Early singing interactions affect musical preferences and facilitate vocabulary building. *Journal of Child Language*, 1–26.

François, C., Chobert, J., Besson, M. & Schön, D. (2013). Music training for the development of speech segmentation. *Cerebral Cortex*, 23(9), 2038–2043. http://doi.org/10.1093/cercor/bhs180.

Frankford, S.A., Heller Murray, E.S., Masapollo, M., Cai, S. *et al.* (2021). The neural circuitry underlying the 'rhythm effect' in stuttering. *Journal of Speech, Language, and Hearing Research*, 64(6S), 2325–2346.

Frischen, U., Schwarzer, G. & Degé, F. (2021). Music lessons enhance executive functions in 6-to 7-year-old children. *Learning and Instruction*, 74, 101442.

Fujii, S. & Wan, C.Y. (2014). The role of rhythm in speech and language rehabilitation: The SEP hypothesis. *Frontiers in Human Neuroscience*, 8, 777.

Fujiwara, K., Kimura, M. & Daibo, I. (2020). Rhythmic features of movement synchrony for bonding individuals in dyadic interaction. *Journal of Nonverbal Behavior*, 44(1), 173–193.

Fusaroli, R., Grossman, R., Bilenberg, N., Cantio, C., Jepsen, J.R.M. & Weed, E. (2021). Toward a cumulative science of vocal markers of autism: A cross-linguistic meta-analysis-based investigation of acoustic markers in American and Danish autistic children. *Autism Research*, 15(4), 653–664.

Garcia-Real, T., Diaz-Roman, T.M., Garcia-Martinez, V. & Vieiro-Iglesias, P. (2013). Clinical and acoustic vocal profile in children with attention deficit hyperactivity disorder. *Journal of Voice*, 27(6), 787.

Gasparini, L., Langus, A., Tsuji, S. & Boll-Avetisyan, N. (2021). Quantifying the role of rhythm in infants' language discrimination abilities: A meta-analysis. *Cognition*, 213, 104757.

Gathercole, S.E. (2006). Nonword repetition and word learning: The nature of the relationship. *Applied Psycholinguistics*, 27(04), 513–543. http://doi.org/10.1017/S0142716406060383.

Georgiadis, P., Iakovidis, P., Trevlakis, M., Xalkia, A. & Tsakona, P. (2019). Respiratory intervention in children 7–14 years old with autism spectrum disorder, attention-deficit/hyperactivity disorder and Down syndrome in special schools in Central Macedonia-Hellas. *International Research Journal of Public and Environmental Health*, 6(8), 191–201.

Gérard, C. & Drake, C. (1990). The inability of young children to reproduce intensity differences in musical rhythms. *Perception & Psychophysics*, 48(1), 91–101.

Getchell, N. & Whitall, J. (2003). How do children coordinate simultaneous upper and lower extremity tasks? The development of dual motor task coordination. *Journal of Experimental Child Psychology*, 85(2), 120–140.

Gick, B. & Stavness, I. (2013). Modularizing speech. *Frontiers in Psychology*, 4, 977.

Gill, S.P. (2012). Rhythmic synchrony and mediated interaction: Towards a framework of rhythm in embodied interaction. *AI & Society*, 27(1), 111–127.

Goble, D.J., Hurvitz, E.A. & Brown, S.H. (2009). Deficits in the ability to use proprioceptive feedback in children with hemiplegic cerebral palsy. *International Journal of Rehabilitation Research*, 32(3), 267–269.

Goffi-Fynn, J.C. & Carroll, L.M. (2013). Collaboration and conquest: MTD as viewed by voice teacher (singing voice specialist) and speech-language pathologist. *Journal of Voice*, 27(3), 391.e9–391.e14.

Gordon, R.L., Fehd, H.M. & McCandliss, B.D. (2015). Does music training enhance literacy skills? A meta-analysis. *Frontiers in Psychology*, 6, 1777.

Goswami, U. (2008). *Mental Capital and Wellbeing: Making the Most of Ourselves in the 21st Century. Learning Difficulties: Future Challenges.* London: Government Office for Science.

Goswami, U. (2011). A temporal sampling framework for developmental dyslexia. *Trends in Cognitive Sciences*, 15(1), 3–10.

Goswami, U. (2012). Entraining the brain: Applications to language research and links to musical entrainment. *Empirical Musicology Review*, 7, 57–63.

Goswami, U. (2019a). A neural oscillations perspective on phonological development and phonological processing in developmental dyslexia. *Language and Linguistics Compass*, 13(5), e12328.

Goswami, U. (2019b). Speech rhythm and language acquisition: An amplitude modulation phase hierarchy perspective. *Annals of the New York Academy of Sciences*, 1453, 67–78. https://doi.org/10.1111/nyas.14137.

Goswami, U. & Leong, V. (2013). Speech rhythm and temporal structure: Converging perspectives? *Laboratory Phonology*, 4(1), 67–92.

Graf, C., Schierz, O., Steinke, H., Körner, A. *et al.* (2019). Sex hormones in association with general joint laxity and hypermobility in the temporomandibular joint in adolescents: Results of the epidemiologic LIFE child study. *Journal of Oral Rehabilitation*, 46(11), 1023–1030.

Grahame, R. (1999). Joint hypermobility and genetic collagen disorders: Are they related? *Arch Dis Child*, 80, 188–191. https://doi.org/10.1136/ adc.80.2.188.

Grahn, J.A. & Schuit, D. (2012). Individual differences in rhythmic ability: Behavioral and neuroimaging investigations. *Psychomusicology: Music, Mind, and Brain*, 22(2), 105.

Groen, M.A., Alku, P. & Bishop, D.V.M. (2008). Lateralisation of auditory processing in Down syndrome: A study of T-complex peaks Ta and Tb. *Biological Psychology*, 79(2), 148–157.

Gutstein, S.E., Burgess, A.F. & Montfort, K. (2007). Evaluation of the relationship development intervention program. *Autism*, 11, 397–411. https://doi.org/10.1177/1362361307079603.

Habibi, A., Damasio, A., Ilari, B., Veiga, R., Joshi, A.A., Leahy, R.M. & Damasio, H. (2018). Childhood music training induces change in micro and macroscopic brain structure: Results from a longitudinal study. *Cerebral Cortex*, 28(12), 4336–4347.

Haesen, B., Boets, B. & Wagemans, J. (2011). A review of behavioural and electrophysiological studies on auditory processing and speech perception in autism spectrum disorders. *Research in Autism Spectrum Disorders*, 5(2), 701–714.

Han, Y.J. (2021). Mediating effect of cognitive load in song learning with visually presented lyrics. *Psychology of Music*, 49(6), 1462–1477.

Hannon, E.E., Lévêque, Y., Nave, K.M. & Trehub, S.E. (2016). Exaggeration of language-specific rhythms in English and French children's songs. *Frontiers in Psychology*, 7, 939.

Hannon, E.E., Soley, G. & Ullal, S. (2012). Familiarity overrides complexity in rhythm perception: A cross-cultural comparison of American and Turkish listeners. *Journal of Experimental Psychology: Human Perception and Performance*, 38(3), 543.

Harris, J.G., Khiani, S.J., Lowe, S.A. & Vora, S.S. (2013). Respiratory symptoms in children with Ehlers-Danlos syndrome. *Journal of Allergy and Clinical Immunology: In Practice*, 1(6), 684–686. https://doi.org/10.1016/j.jaip.2013.06.008.

Haslbeck, F.B. & Bassler, D. (2018). Music from the very beginning: A neuroscience-based framework for music as therapy for preterm infants and their parents. *Frontiers in Behavioral Neuroscience*, 12, 112.

Hengen, J., Hammarström, I.L. & Stenfelt, S. (2018). Perceived voice quality and voice-related problems among older adults with hearing impairments. *Journal of Speech, Language, and Hearing Research*, 61(9), 2168–2178.

Hidalgo, C., Falk, S. & Schön, D. (2017). Speak on time! Effects of a musical rhythmic training on children with hearing loss. *Hearing Research*, 351, 11–18.

Hillier, A., Kopec, J., Poto, N., Tivarus, M. & Beversdorf, D.Q. (2016). Increased physiological responsiveness to preferred music among young adults with autism spectrum disorders. *Psychology of Music*, 44(3), 481–492.

Hirano, M. & Kakita, Y. (1985). Cover-Body Theory of Vocal Fold Vibration. In R.G. Daniloff (ed.), *Speech Science: Recent Advances*, pp.1–46. San Diego, CA: College-Hill Press.

Hocevar-Boltezar, I., Radsel, Z., Vatovec, J., Geczy, B. *et al.* (2006). Change of phonation control after cochlear implantation. *Otology & Neurotology*, 27(4), 499–503.

Hodges, P.W., Butler, J.E., McKenzie, D.K. & Gandevia, S.C. (1997). Contraction of the human diaphragm during rapid postural adjustments. *The Journal of Physiology*, 505(Pt 2), 539.

Hodges, P.W., Eriksson, A.M., Shirley, D. & Gandevia, S.C. (2005). Intra-abdominal pressure increases stiffness of the lumbar spine. *Journal of Biomechanics*, 38(9), 1873–1880.

Hodges, P.W., Sapsford, R. & Pengel, L.H.M. (2007). Postural and respiratory functions of the pelvic floor muscles. *Neurourology and Urodynamics*, 26(3), 362–371.

Honda, K. (1983). Relationship between pitch control and vowel articulation. *Haskins Laboratories Status Report on Speech Research*, 73, 269–282.

Honing, H. (2019) *The Evolving Animal Orchestra: In Search of What Makes Us Musical*. Cambridge, MA: MIT Press.

Horne, R.S., Wijayaratne, P., Nixon, G.M. & Walter, L.M. (2019). Sleep and sleep disordered breathing in children with Down syndrome: Effects on behaviour, neurocognition and the cardiovascular system. *Sleep Medicine Reviews*, 44, 1–11.

Horowitz, S.S. (2012). *The Universal Sense: How Hearing Shapes the Mind*. New York, NY: Bloomsbury Publishing.

Houlahan, M. & Tacka, P. (2015). *Kodály Today: A Cognitive Approach to Elementary Music Education*. Oxford University Press.

Hunter, A., Morgan, A.W. & Bird, H.A. (1998). A survey of Ehlers-Danlos syndrome: Hearing, voice, speech and swallowing difficulties. Is there an underlying relationship? *British Journal of Rheumatology*, 37(7), 803–804.

Ilari, B.S., Keller, P., Damasio, H. & Habibi, A. (2016). The development of musical skills of underprivileged children over the course of 1 year: A study in the context of an El Sistema-inspired program. *Frontiers in Psychology*, 7, 62.

Ilari, B., Fesjian, C. & Habibi, A. (2018). Entrainment, theory of mind, and prosociality in child musicians. *Music & Science*, 1, 2059204317753153.

Jackson, S.A., Treharne, D.A. & Boucher, J. (1997). Rhythm and language in children with moderate learning difficulties. *European Journal of Disorders of Communication*, 32(1), 99–108.

Jamey, K., Foster, N.E., Sharda, M., Tuerk, C., Nadig, A. & Hyde, K.L. (2019). Evidence for intact melodic and rhythmic perception in children with autism spectrum disorder. *Research in Autism Spectrum Disorders*, 64, 1–12.

Janzen, T.B. & Thaut, M.H. (2018). Rethinking the role of music in the neurodevelopment of autism spectrum disorder. *Music & Science*, 1, 2059204318769639.

Jarvis, E.D. (2007). Neural systems for vocal learning in birds and humans: A synopsis. *Journal of Ornithology*, 148(1), 35–44.

Jeffery, T. (2016). Speaking in Harmony: An Exploration of the Potential for Rhythm and Song to Support Speech Production in Four Young Adults with Down Syndrome. Doctoral dissertation, University of Sheffield.

Jeffery, T., Cunningham, S. & Whiteside, S.P. (2018). Analyses of sustained vowels in Down syndrome (DS): A case study using spectrograms and perturbation data to investigate voice quality in four adults with DS. *Journal of Voice*, 32(5), 644.e11–644.e24.

Jeffery, T., Postăvaru, G., Matei, R. & Meizel, K. (2021). 'I have had to stop singing because I can't take the pain': Experiences of voice, ability, and loss in singers with hypermobility spectrum disorders. *Journal of Voice*. doi: 10.1016/j.jvoice.2021.11.017.

Jeffries, K.J., Fritz, J.B. & Braun, A.R. (2003). Words in melody: An H215O PET study of brain activation during singing and speaking. *Neuroreport*, 14(5), 749–754.

Jentschke, S. (2016). The Relationship between Music and Language. In S. Hallam, I. Cross & M. Thaut (eds), *The Oxford Handbook of Music Psychology*, pp.343–355. Oxford: Oxford University Press.

Johnstone, T. & Scherer, K.R. (1999, August). The Effects of Emotions on Voice Quality. In *Proceedings of the XIVth International Congress of Phonetic Sciences* (pp.2029–2032). Department of Linguistics, University of California at Berkeley, California.

Jovanov, E. & Maxfield, M.C. (2011). Entraining the Brain and Body. In J. Berger & G. Turow (eds), *Music, Science and the Rhythmic Brain: Cultural and Clinical Implications*, pp.31–48. New York, NY: Routledge.

Kalashnikova, M., Peter, V., Di Liberto, G.M., Lalor, E.C. & Burnham, D. (2018). Infant-directed speech facilitates seven-month-old infants' cortical tracking of speech. *Scientific Reports*, 8(1), 1–8.

Kalender, B., Trehub, S.E. & Schellenberg, E.G. (2013). Cross-cultural differences in meter perception. *Psychological Research*, 77(2), 196–203.

Kargas, N., López, B., Morris, P. & Reddy, V. (2016). Relations among detection of syllable stress, speech abnormalities, and communicative ability in adults with autism spectrum disorders. *Journal of Speech, Language, and Hearing Research*, 59(2), 206–215.

Katz, J.J., Ando, M. & Wiseheart, M. (2021). Optimizing song retention through the spacing effect. *Cognitive Research: Principles and Implications*, 6(1), 1–17.

Kayes, G. & Fisher, J. (2016). *This Is a Voice: 99 Exercises to Train, Project and Harness the Power of Your Voice*. London: Wellcome Collection.

Keles, M.N., Elbasan, B., Apaydin, U., Aribas, Z., Bakirtas, A. & Kokturk, N. (2018). Effects of inspiratory muscle training in children with cerebral palsy: A randomized controlled trial. *Brazilian Journal of Physical Therapy*, 22(6), 493–501.

Kent, R.D. & Vorperian, H.K. (2013). Speech impairment in Down syndrome: A review. *Journal of Speech, Language, and Hearing Research*, 56, 178–210. http://doi.org/10.1044/1092-4388(2012/12-0148.

Key, A.P. & D'Ambrose, S.K. (2021). Speech processing in autism spectrum disorder: An integrative review of auditory neurophysiology findings. *Journal of Speech, Language, and Hearing Research*, 64(11), 4192–4212. https://doi.org/10.1044/2021_JSLHR-20-00738.

Kirby, M.L. & Burland, K. (2022). Exploring the functions of music in the lives of young people on the autism spectrum. *Psychology of Music*, 50(2), 562–578. https://doi.org/10.1177/03057356211008968.

Koelsch, S. (2014). Brain correlates of music-evoked emotions. *Nature Reviews Neuroscience*, 15(3), 170–180.

Kolinsky, R., Lidji, P., Peretz, I., Besson, M. & Morais, J. (2009). Processing interactions between phonology and melody: Vowels sing but consonants speak. *Cognition*, 112(1), 1–20.

Koseki, T., Kakizaki, F., Hayashi, S., Nishida, N. & Itoh, M. (2019). Effect of forward head posture on thoracic shape and respiratory function. *Journal of Physical Therapy Science*, 31(1), 63–68.

Kösem, A., Bosker, H.R., Takashima, A., Meyer, A., Jensen, O. & Hagoort, P. (2018). Neural entrainment determines the words we hear. *Current Biology*, 28(18), 2867–2875.

Kraus, N. & Chandrasekaran, B. (2010). Music training for the development of auditory skills. *Nature Reviews Neuroscience*, 11(8), 599–605. http://doi.org/10.1038/nrn2882.

Krishnamurthy, R. & Ramani, S.A. (2020). Aerodynamic and acoustic characteristics of voice in children with Down syndrome – A systematic review. *International Journal of Pediatric Otorhinolaryngology*, 133, 109946.

Kryshtopava, M., Van Lierde, K., Meerschman, I., D'Haeseleer, E. *et al.* (2017). Brain activity during phonation in women with muscle tension dysphonia: An fMRI study. *Journal of Voice*, 31(6), 675–690. doi: 10.1016/j.jvoice.2017.03.010.

Kuang, J. (2017). Covariation between voice quality and pitch: Revisiting the case of Mandarin creaky voice. *The Journal of the Acoustical Society of America*, 142(3), 1693–1706.

Ladányi, E., Persici, V., Fiveash, A., Tillmann, B. & Gordon, R.L. (2020). Is atypical rhythm a risk factor for developmental speech and language disorders? *Wiley Interdisciplinary Reviews: Cognitive Science*, 11(5), e1528.

LaGasse, A.B. & Hardy, M.W. (2013). Rhythm, movement, and autism: Using rhythmic rehabilitation research as a model for autism. *Frontiers in Integrative Neuroscience*, 7, 19.

Large, E.W., Herrera, J.A. & Velasco, M.J. (2015). Neural networks for beat perception in musical rhythm. *Frontiers in Systems Neuroscience*, 9, 159.

Laver, J. (1980). *The Phonetic Description of Voice Quality*. Cambridge: Cambridge University Press.

Lecanuet, J.P. & Schaal, B. (2002). Sensory performances in the human foetus: A brief summary of research. *Intellectica*, 34(1), 29–56.

Lechien, J.R., Saussez, S., Nacci, A., Barillari, M.R. *et al.* (2019). Association between laryngopharyngeal reflux and benign vocal folds lesions: A systematic review. *The Laryngoscope*, 129(9), E329–E341.

Lee, L.J., Chang, A.T., Coppieters, M.W. & Hodges, P.W. (2010). Changes in sitting posture induce multiplanar changes in chest wall shape and motion with breathing. *Respiratory Physiology & Neurobiology*, 170(3), 236–245.

Lee, M.T., Thorpe, J. & Verhoeven, J. (2009). Intonation and phonation in young adults with Down syndrome. *Journal of Voice*, 23(1), 82–87.

Lenneberg, E.H. (1967). The biological foundations of language. *Hospital Practice*, 2(12), 59–67.

Leong, V. & Goswami, U. (2014). Assessment of rhythmic entrainment at multiple timescales in dyslexia: Evidence for disruption to syllable timing. *Hearing Research*, 308, 141–161.

Lerens, E., Araneda, R., Renier, L. & De Volder, A.G. (2014). Improved beat asynchrony detection in early blind individuals. *Perception*, 43(10), 1083–1096.

Levin, I., Lewek, M.D., Feasel, J. & Thorpe, D.E. (2017). Gait training with visual feedback and proprioceptive input to reduce gait asymmetry in adults with cerebral palsy: A case series. *Pediatric Physical Therapy*, 29(2), 138–145.

Levitin, D.J. (2006). *This is Your Brain on Music: The Science of a Human Obsession*. New York, NY: Penguin.

Levitin, D.J. (2019). Medicine's melodies: Music, health and well-being. *Music and Medicine*, 11(4), 236–244.

Lidji, P., Jolicœur, P., Kolinsky, R., Moreau, P., Connolly, J.F. & Peretz, I. (2010). Early integration of vowel and pitch processing: A mismatch negativity study. *Clinical Neurophysiology*, 121(4), 533–541.

Lindley-Baker, J. & Mills, L. (2022). Playing to learn: Learning to TALK. *British Journal of Special Education*, 49(3), 350–374. https://doi.org/10.1111/1467-8578.12411.

Lloyd, P. (2007). *Let's All Listen. Songs for Group Work in Settings that Include Students with Learning Difficulties and Autism*. London: Jessica Kingsley Publishers.

Loehr, D. (2007). Aspects of rhythm in gesture and speech. *Gesture*, 7(2), 179–214.

Loewy, J.V. (1995). The musical stages of speech: A developmental model of pre-verbal sound making. *Music Therapy*, 13(1), 47–73.

Loney, N. & Adams, M. (2018). *Vocal Warm-ups and Technical Exercises for Kids*. Hemford, Ontario: Full Voice Music.

Ludlow, C.L. & Loucks, T. (2003). Stuttering: A dynamic motor control disorder. *Journal of Fluency Disorders*, 28(4), 273–295. http://doi.org/10.1016/j.jfludis.2003.07.001.

Ma, W., Golinkoff, R.M., Houston, D.M. & Hirsh-Pasek, K. (2011). Word learning in infant- and adult-directed speech. *Language Learning and Development*, 7(3), 185–201.

MacDonald, R., Kreutz, G. & Mitchell, L. (eds) (2013). *Music, Health, and Wellbeing*. Oxford: Oxford University Press.

MacDonald, R.A., O'Donnell, P.J. & Davies, J. (1999). An empirical investigation into the effects of structured music workshops for individuals with intellectual disabilities. *Journal of Applied Research in Intellectual Disabilities*, 12(3), 225–240.

McCallion, M. (1998). *The Voice Book*. London: Faber & Faber.

Mainka, S. & Mallien, G. (2014). Rhythmic Speech Cueing (RSC). In M.H. Thaut & V. Hoemberg (eds), *Handbook of Neurologic Music Therapy*, pp.150–160. Oxford: Oxford University Press.

Malloch, S. & Trevarthen, C. (2018). The human nature of music. *Frontiers in Psychology*, 9, 1680.

Marcell, M. (1995). Relationships between hearing and auditory cognition in Down syndrome youth. *Down Syndrome Research and Practice*, 3(3), 75–91. http://doi.org/10.3104/reports.54.

Margulis, E.H., Simchy-Gross, R. & Black, J.L. (2015). Pronunciation difficulty, temporal regularity, and the speech-to-song illusion. *Frontiers in Psychology*, 6, 48.

Marom, M.K., Gilboa, A. & Bodner, E. (2018). Musical features and interactional functions of echolalia in children with autism within the music therapy dyad. *Nordic Journal of Music Therapy*, 27(3), 175–196.

Martins, M., Neves, L., Rodrigues, P., Vasconcelos, O. & Castro, S.L. (2018). Orff-based music training enhances children's manual dexterity and bimanual coordination. *Frontiers in Psychology*, 9, 2616.

Marx, I., Cortese, S., Koelch, M.G. & Hacker, T. (2021). Meta-analysis: Altered perceptual timing abilities in attention-deficit/hyperactivity disorder. *Journal of the American Academy of Child & Adolescent Psychiatry*, 61(7), 866–880.

Masala, K.S. & Presence, C. (2004). *Rhythm Play! Rhythm Activities and Initiatives for Adults, Facilitators, Teachers, & Kids!* Denver, CO: FUNdoing Publications.

Mason-Apps, E., Stojanovic, V. & Houston-Price, C. (2011). Early word segmentation in typically developing infants and infants with Down syndrome: A preliminary study. In *Proceedings of the 17th International Congress of Phonetic Sciences* (pp.1334–1337).

Mathur, R.P. & Banik, A. (2015). A comparative study of voice characteristics of adults with hearing impairment amplified at different ages and normal hearing. *International Journal of Multidisciplinary Research and Development*, 2(11), 507–511.

Matsubara, M., Terasawa, H. & Hiraga, R. (2014). The effect of musical experience on rhythm perception for hearing-impaired undergraduates. In *2014 IEEE International Conference on Systems, Man and Cybernetics* (pp.1666–1669). IEEE.

Matsuyama, K. (2005). Correlation between musical responsiveness and developmental age among early age children as assessed by the Non-Verbal Measurement of the Musical Responsiveness of Children. *Medical Science Monitor: International Medical Journal of Experimental and Clinical Research*, 11(10), CR485–492.

Mayo, O. & Gordon, I. (2020). In and out of synchrony: Behavioral and physiological dynamics of dyadic interpersonal coordination. *Psychophysiology*, 57(6), e13574.

McCabe, P., Rosenthal, J.B. & McLeod, S. (1998). Features of developmental dyspraxia in the general speech-impaired population? *Clinical Linguistics & Phonetics*, 12(2), 105–126.

McPherson, G. (ed). (2015). *The Child as Musician: A Handbook of Musical Development*. Oxford: Oxford University Press.

Mehler, J., Jusczyk, P., Lambertz, G., Halsted, N., Bertoncini, J. & Amiel-Tison, C. (1988). *A precursor of language acquisition in young infants. Cognition*, 29(2), 143–178.

Merchant, H. & Honing, H. (2014). Are non-human primates capable of rhythmic entrainment? Evidence for the gradual audiomotor evolution hypothesis. *Frontiers in Neuroscience*, 7, 274.

Merker, B.H., Madison, G.S. & Eckerdal, P. (2009). On the role and origin of isochrony in human rhythmic entrainment. *Cortex*, 45(1), 4–17.

Miendlarzewska, E.A. & Trost, W.J. (2014). How musical training affects cognitive development: Rhythm, reward and other modulating variables. *Frontiers in Neuroscience*, 7, 279.

Miller, D., Rees, J. & Pearson, A. (2021). 'Masking is life': Experiences of masking in autistic and nonautistic adults. *Autism in Adulthood*, 3(4), 330–338.

Ming, X., Patel, R., Kang, V., Chokroverty, S. & Julu, P.O. (2016). Respiratory and autonomic dysfunction in children with autism spectrum disorders. *Brain and Development*, 38(2), 225–232.

Mitchell, R.B., Call, E. & Kelly, J. (2003). Ear, nose and throat disorders in children with Down syndrome. *The Laryngoscope*, 113(2), 259–263.

Mithen, S. (2005). *The Singing Neanderthals*. London: Weidenfeld & Nicholson.

Montirosso, R. & McGlone, F. (2020). The body comes first. Embodied reparation and the co-creation of infant bodily-self. *Neuroscience & Biobehavioral Reviews*, 113, 77–87.

Moodley, D.T., Swanepoel, C., Van Lierde, K., Abdoola, S. & Van der Linde, J. (2019). Vocal characteristics of school-aged children with and without attention deficit hyperactivity disorder. *Journal of Voice*, 33(6), 945.

Morgan, A.W., Pearson, S.B., Davies, S., Gooi, H.C. & Bird, H.A. (2007). Asthma and airways collapse in two heritable disorders of connective tissue. *Annals of the Rheumatic Diseases*, 66(10), 1369–1373. https://doi.org/10.1136/ard.2006.062224.

Moro, A. (2016). *Impossible Languages*. Cambridge, MA: MIT Press.

Moura, C.P., Cunha, L.M., Vilarinho, H., Cunha, M.J. *et al.* (2008). Voice parameters in children with Down syndrome. *Journal of Voice*, 22(1), 34–42.

Mulvey, G. (2007). Handedness and Verbal Motor Integration in Adults with Down Syndrome (Order No. 3270607). Available from ProQuest Central (304896363): www.proquest.com/dissertations-theses/handedness-verbal-motor-integration-adults-with/docview/304896363/se-2.

Nakano, T., Kato, N. & Kitazawa, S. (2011). Lack of eyeblink entrainments in autism spectrum disorders. *Neuropsychologia*, 49(9), 2784–2790.

Nazzi, T., Bertoncini, J. & Mehler, J. (1998). Language discrimination by newborns: Toward an understanding of the role of rhythm. *Journal of Experimental Psychology: Human Perception and Performance*, 24(3), 756.

Nazzi, T. & Ramus, F. (2003). Perception and acquisition of linguistic rhythm by infants. *Speech Communication*, 41(1), 233–243.

Ngan, A., Hand, L., May, D., Antipova, E. & Purdy, S. (2011). Social communication intervention for children with autism spectrum disorders: Background and teacher strategies in an experience sharing program. *New Zealand Journal of Speech Language Therapy*, 66, 46–65.

Nicholls, C. (2014). *Body, Breath and Being: A New Guide to the Alexander Technique*. Hove: D&B Publishing.

Nielsen, M. (2017). ADHD and temporality: A desynchronized way of being in the world. *Medical Anthropology*, 36(3), 260–272.

Nind, M. & Hewett, D. (1994) *Access to Communication: Developing the Basics of Communication with People with Severe Learning Difficulties through Intensive Interaction*. London: David Fulton.

Nind, M. & Powell, S. (2000). Intensive interaction and autism: Some theoretical concerns. *Children & Society*, 14(2), 98–109.

Nip, I.S. & Garellek, M. (2021). Voice quality of children with cerebral palsy. *Journal of Speech, Language, and Hearing Research*, 64(8), 3051–3059.

Nketia, J.K. (1974). *The Music of Africa*. New York, NY: W.W. Norton.

Nooteboom, S. (1997). The prosody of speech: Melody and rhythm. *The Handbook of Phonetic Sciences*, 5, 640–673.

Novembre, G. & Keller, P.E. (2014). A conceptual review on action-perception coupling in the musicians' brain: What is it good for? *Frontiers in Human Neuroscience*, 8, 603.

Nunes-Silva, M., Caetano, A.A.R., Alves, S.O. & de Mello, G.T. (2018). Evaluation of Music Cognition in Children and Adolescents with Attention-Deficit/Hyperactivity Disorder. *Proceedings of the 11th International Conference of Students of Systematic Musicology*, Brazil, pp.88–93: https://www.researchgate.net/publication/329104764_Evaluation_of_music_cognition_in_children_and_adolescents_with_Attention-Deficit_Hyperactivity_Disorder

O'Connor, K. (2012). Auditory processing in autism spectrum disorder: A review. *Neuroscience & Biobehavioral Reviews*, 36(2), 836–854.

Ockelford, A. (2008). *Music for Children and Young People with Complex Needs*. Oxford: Oxford University Press.

Ockelford, A., Welch, G., Jewell-Gore, L., Cheng, E., Vogiatzoglou, A. & Himonides, E. (2011). Phase 2: Gauging the music development of children with complex needs. *European Journal of Special Needs Education*, 26(2), 177–199. http://doi.org/10.1080/08856257.2011.563606.

Ockelford, A. (2013). *Music, Language and Autism: Exceptional Strategies for Exceptional Minds*. London: Jessica Kingsley Publishers.

Ockelford, A. (2016). Prodigious Musical Talent in Blind Children with Autism and Learning Difficulties: Interpretations from Psychology, Education, Musicology, and Ethnomusicology. In G.E. McPherson (ed.), *Musical Prodigies: Interpretations from Psychology, Education, Musicology, and Ethnomusicology*. Oxford: Oxford University Press.

Ockelford, A. (2018). *Tuning In Music Book: Sixty-four Songs for Children with Complex Needs and Visual Impairment to Promote Language, Social Interaction and Wider Development*. London: Jessica Kingsley Publishers.

Onyiuke, Y.S. (2005). Childhood Music Education in Nigeria: A Case Study. DMus Dissertation. University of Pretoria.

Ogawa, M., Hosokawa, K., Yoshida, M., Yoshii, T., Shiromoto, O. & Inohara, H. (2013). Immediate effectiveness of humming on the supraglottic compression in subjects with muscle tension dysphonia. *Folia Phoniatrica et Logopaedica*, 65(3), 123–128.

Okuro, R.T., Morcillo, A.M., Ribeiro, M.Â., Sakano, E., Conti, P.B. & Ribeiro, J.D. (2011). Mouth breathing and forward head posture: Effects on respiratory bio-mechanics and exercise capacity in children. *Brasilian Journal of Pulmonology*, 37(4), 471–479.

Ott, P. (2011). *Music for Special Kids: Musical Activities, Songs, Instruments and Resources*. London: Jessica Kingsley Publishers.

Pandit, C. & Fitzgerald, D.A. (2012). Respiratory problems in children with Down syndrome. *Journal of Paediatrics and Child Health*, 48(3), E147–E152.

Papatzikis, E. (2017). The educational neuroscience perspective of ABR and lull-abies: Setting up an infants brain development study. *International Journal of Cross Disciplinary Subjects in Education*, 8, 3179–3185.

Parbery-Clark, A., Anderson, S., Hittner, E. & Kraus, N. (2012). Musical experience strengthens the neural representation of sounds important for communica-tion in middle-aged adults. *Frontiers in Aging Neuroscience*, 4, 30.

Parncutt, R. (2016). Prenatal Development. In G.E. McPherson (ed.), *The Child as Musician: A Handbook of Musical Development*, second edition, pp.1–31. Oxford: Oxford University Press.

Patel, A.D. (2003). Rhythm in language and music: Parallels and differences. *Annals of the New York Academy of Sciences*, 999(1), 140–143.

Patel, A.D. (2008). *Music, Language, and the Brain*. Oxford: Oxford University Press.

Patel, A.D. (2011). Why would musical training benefit the neural encoding of speech? The OPERA hypothesis. *Frontiers in Psychology*, 2, 142.

Patel, A.D. (2014). Can nonlinguistic musical training change the way the brain processes speech? The expanded OPERA hypothesis. *Hearing Research*, 308, 98–108.

Patel, A.D. (2021). Vocal learning as a preadaptation for the evolution of human beat perception and synchronization. *Philosophical Transactions of the Royal Society*, B, 376(1835), 20200326.

Patel, S.P., Kim, J.H., Larson, C.R. & Losh, M. (2019). Mechanisms of voice con-trol related to prosody in autism spectrum disorder and first-degree rela-tives. *Autism Research*, 12(8), 1192–1210.

Pavão, S.L. & Rocha, N.A.C.F. (2017). Sensory processing disorders in children with cerebral palsy. *Infant Behavior and Development*, 46, 1–6.

Pearson, A. & Hodgetts, S. (2020). Can cerebral lateralisation explain heterogene-ity in language and increased non-right handedness in autism? A literature review. *Research in Developmental Disabilities*, 105, 103738.

Pearson, A. & Rose, K. (2021). A conceptual analysis of autistic masking: Under-standing the narrative of stigma and the illusion of choice. *Autism in Adult-hood*, 3(1), 52–60.

Pennington, L., Lombardo, E., Steen, N. & Miller, N. (2018). Acoustic changes in the speech of children with cerebral palsy following an intensive program of dysarthria therapy. *International Journal of Language & Communication Disorders*, 53(1), 182–195.

Perin, C., Valagussa, G., Mazzucchelli, M., Gariboldi, V. *et al.* (2020). Physiolog-ical profile assessment of posture in children and adolescents with autism spectrum disorder and typically developing peers. *Brain Sciences,* 10(10), 681.

Perkins, R., Ascenso, S., Atkins, L., Fancourt, D. & Williamon, A. (2016). Making music for mental health: How group drumming mediates recovery. *Psychology of Well-being*, 6(1), 1–17.

Perkins, R., Mason-Bertrand, A., Fancourt, D., Baxter, L. & Williamon, A. (2020). How participatory music engagement supports mental well-being: A meta-ethnography. *Qualitative Health Research*, 30(12), 1924–1940.

Perry, M.M.R. (2003). Relating improvisational music therapy with severely and multiply disabled children to communication development. *Journal of Music Therapy*, 40(3), 227–246.

Peter, B. & Stoel-Gammon, C. (2008). Central timing deficits in subtypes of primary speech disorders. *Clinical Linguistics & Phonetics*, 22(3), 171–198.

Pettinato, M. & Verhoeven, J. (2009). Production and perception of word stress in children and adolescents with Down syndrome. *Down Syndrome Research and Practice*, 1–13.

Phillips, K. (2003). *Teaching Kids to Sing*. New York, NY: Schirmer.

Phillips-Silver, J. (2009). On the meaning of movement in music, development and the brain. *Contemporary Music Review*, 28(3), 293–314.

Phillips-Silver, J. & Trainor, L.J. (2005). Feeling the beat: movement influences infant rhythm perception. *Science*, 308(5727), 1430–1430.

Phillips-Silver, J. & Trainor, L.J. (2007). Hearing what the body feels: Auditory encoding of rhythmic movement. *Cognition*, 105(3), 533–546.

Picard, B.M. (2009). Music and Down's Syndrome. Unpublished master's thesis'. Royal Welsh College of Music and Drama, Cardiff, Wales.

Pryce, M. (1994). The voice of people with Down yndrome: An EMG biofeedback study. *Down Syndrome Research and Practice*, 2(3), 106–111.

Racette, A. & Peretz, I. (2007). Learning lyrics: To sing or not to sing? *Memory & Cognition*, 35(2), 242–253.

Rajendran, V., Roy, F.G. & Jeevanantham, D. (2012). Postural control, motor skills, and health-related quality of life in children with hearing impairment: A systematic review. *European Archives of Oto-Rhino-Laryngology*, 269(4), 1063–1071.

Ramey, M. (2011). *Group Music Activities for Adults with Intellectual and Developmental Disabilities*. London: Jessica Kingsley Publishers.

Ramia, M., Musharrafieh, U., Khaddage, W. & Sabri, A. (2014). Revisiting Down syndrome from the ENT perspective: Review of literature and recommendations. *European Archives of Oto-Rhino-Laryngology*, 271(5), 863–869.

Ramos, J.S., Feniman, M.R., Gielow, I. & Silverio, K.C.A. (2018). Correlation between voice and auditory processing. *Journal of Voice*, 32(6), 771 .e25–771.e36.

Remington, A. & Fairnie, J. (2017). A sound advantage: Increased auditory capacity in autism. *Cognition*, 166, 459–465.

Repp, B.H. & Doggett, R. (2007). Tapping to a very slow beat: A comparison of musicians and nonmusicians. *Music Perception: An Interdisciplinary Journal*, 24(4), 367–376.

Repp, B.H. & Su, Y.-H. (2013). Sensorimotor synchronization: A review of recent research (2006–2012). *Psychonomic Bulletin & Review*, 20(3), 403–452. http://doi.org/10.3758/s13423-012-0371-2.

Riccio, C.A., Hynd, G.W., Cohen, M.J., Hall, J. & Molt, L. (1994). Comorbidity of central auditory processing disorder and attention-deficit hyperactivity disorder. *Journal of the American Academy of Child & Adolescent Psychiatry*, 33(6), 849–857.

Ridgway, R. (2013). Giving a Voice to the Hard to Reach: Song as an Effective Medium for Communicating with PMLD Children Who Have Low Social Tolerance. Doctoral dissertation, Durham University.

Rimmer, J., Giddings, C.E.B., Cavalli, L. & Hartley, B.E.J. (2008). Dysphonia: A rare early symptom of Ehlers-Danlos syndrome? *International Journal of Pediatric Otorhinolaryngology*, 72(12), 1889–1892. https://doi.org/10.1016/j.ijporl.2008.09.018.

Rimrodt, S.L. & Johnston, M.V. (2009). Neuronal Plasticity and Developmental Disabilities. In M. Shevell (ed.), *Neurodevelopmental Disabilities: Clinical and Scientific Foundations*, pp.225–240. London: Mac Keith Press.

Ringenbach, S.D., Allen, H., Chung, S. & Jung, M.L. (2006). Specific instructions are important for continuous bimanual drumming in adults with Down syndrome. *Downs Syndrome Research and Practice*, 11(1), 29–36.

Ringenbach, S.D., Mulvey, G.M., Chen, C.C. & Jung, M.L. (2012). Unimanual and bimanual continuous movements benefit from visual instructions in persons with Down syndrome. *Journal of Motor Behavior*, 44(4), 233–239.

Rinta, T. (2008). Potential use of singing in educational settings with pre-pubertal children possessing speech and voice disorders: A psychological perspective. *British Journal of Music Education*, 25(2), 139–158.

Rinta, T. & Welch, G.F. (2008). Should singing activities be included in speech and voice therapy for prepubertal children? *Journal of Voice*, 22(1), 100–112.

Robledo, J., Donnellan, A.M. & Strandt-Conroy, K. (2012). An exploration of sensory and movement differences from the perspective of individuals with autism. *Frontiers in Integrative Neuroscience*, 6, 107.

Roche, R., Viswanathan, P., Clark, J.E. & Whitall, J. (2016). Children with developmental coordination disorder (DCD) can adapt to perceptible and subliminal rhythm changes but are more variable. *Human Movement Science*, 50, 19–29.

Rochette, F., Moussard, A. & Bigand, E. (2014). Music lessons improve auditory perceptual and cognitive performance in deaf children. *Frontiers in Human Neuroscience*, 8.

Rodrigues, M., Nunes, J., Figueiredo, S., Martins de Campos, A. & Geraldo, A.F. (2019). Neuroimaging assessment in Down syndrome: A pictorial review. *Insights into Imaging*, 10(1), 1–13.

Rutkowski, J. (1997). The Nature of Children's Singing Voices: Characteristics and Assessment. In B.A. Roberts (ed.), *The Phenomenon of Singing*, pp.201–209. St. John's, NF: Memorial University Press.

Rutkowski, S., Adamczyk, M., Pastuła, A., Gos, E., Luque-Moreno, C. & Rutkowska, A. (2021). Training using a commercial immersive virtual reality system on hand–eye coordination and reaction time in young musicians: A pilot study. *International Journal of Environmental Research and Public Health*, 18(3), 1297.

Sacks, B. & Buckley, S. (2003). *Motor Development for Individuals with Down Syndrome: An Overview*. Kirkby Lonsdale, Cumbria: Down Syndrome Education Enterprises.

Sacks, O. (2007). *Musicophilia: Tales of Music and the Brain*. London: Picador.

Sacks, O. (2010). *Musicophilia: Tales of Music and the Brain*. Toronto: Vintage Canada.

Safi, F.A., Alyosif, M.A., Imam, S. & Assaly, R.A. (2017). Arytenoid prolapse in 3 patients with Ehler-Danlos syndrome leading to respiratory compromise. *Mayo Clinic Proceedings*, 92(5), 851–853.

Salihović, N., Junuzović-žunić, L., Ibrahimagić, A. & Beganović, L. (2009). Characteristics of voice in stuttering children. *Acta Medica Saliniana*, 38(2), 67–75.

Sapp, W. (2011). Somebody's jumping on the floor: Incorporating music into orientation and mobility for preschoolers with visual impairments. *Journal of Visual Impairment & Blindness*, 105(10), 715–719.

Sapsford, R.R., Richardson, C.A., Maher, C.F. & Hodges, P.W. (2008). Pelvic floor muscle activity in different sitting postures in continent and incontinent women. *Archives of Physical Medicine and Rehabilitation*, 89(9), 1741–1747.

Sataloff, R.T. (2017). *Treatment of Voice Disorders*. San Diego, CA: Plural Publishing.

Saxena, S., Cinar, E., Majnemer, A. & Gagnon, I. (2017). Does dual tasking ability change with age across childhood and adolescence? A systematic scoping review. *International Journal of Developmental Neuroscience*, 58, 35–49.

Schäfer, T., Huron, D., Shanahan, D. & Sedlmeier, P. (2015). The sounds of safety: Stress and danger in music perception. *Frontiers in Psychology*, 6, 1140. https://doi.org/10.3389/fpsyg.2015.01140.

Schlaug, G., Marchina, S. & Norton, A. (2008). From singing to speaking: Why singing may lead to recovery of expressive language function in patients with Broca's aphasia. *Music Perception*, 25(4), 315–323.

Schleuter, S.L. & Schleuter, L.J. (1989). The relationship of rhythm response tasks and PMMA scores with music training, grade level, and sex among K-3 students. *Bulletin of the Council for Research in Music Education*, 1–13.

Schölderle, T., Haas, E., Baumeister, S. & Ziegler, W. (2021). Intelligibility, articulation rate, fluency, and communicative efficiency in typically developing children. *Journal of Speech, Language, and Hearing Research*, 64(7), 2575–2585.

Schön, D. & Tillmann, B. (2015). Short- and long-term rhythmic interventions: Perspectives for language rehabilitation. *Annals of the New York Academy of Sciences*, 1337(1), 32–39.

Schön, D., Boyer, M., Moreno, S., Besson, M., Peretz, I. & Kolinsky, R. (2008). Songs as an aid for language acquisition. *Cognition*, 106(2), 975–983.

Seifart, F., Meyer, J., Grawunder, S. & Dentel, L. (2018). Reducing language to rhythm: Amazonian Bora drummed language exploits speech rhythm for long-distance communication. *Royal Society Open Science*, 5(4), 170354.

Seligman, M.E. (2012). *Flourish: A Visionary New Understanding of Happiness and Well-Being*. New York, NY: Simon and Schuster.

Sheinkopf, S.J., Iverson, J.M., Rinaldi, M.L. & Lester, B.M. (2012). Atypical cry acoustics in 6-month-old infants at risk for autism spectrum disorder. *Autism Research*, 5(5), 331–339.

Sheinkopf, S.J., Mundy, P., Oller, D.K. & Steffens, M. (2000). Vocal atypicalities of preverbal autistic children. *Journal of Autism and Developmental Disorders*, 30(4), 345–354.

Shields, N. (2021). Physiotherapy management of Down syndrome. *Journal of Physiotherapy*, 67(4), 243–251.

Shih, L.C., Piel, J., Warren, A., Kraics, L. *et al.* (2012). Singing in groups for Parkinson's disease (SING-PD): A pilot study of group singing therapy for PD-related voice/speech disorders. *Parkinsonism & Related Disorders*, 18(5), 548–552.

Shriberg, L.D., Paul, R., McSweeny, J.L., Klin, A., Cohen, D.J. & Volkmar, F.R. (2001). Speech and prosody characteristics of adolescents and adults with high-functioning autism and Asperger syndrome. *Journal of Speech, Language, and Hearing Research*, 44(5), 1097–1115.

Simberg, S. & Laine, A. (2007). The resonance tube method in voice therapy: Description and practical implementations. *Logopedics Phoniatrics Vocology*, 32(4), 165–170.

Slater, J., Ashley, R., Tierney, A. & Kraus, N. (2018). Got rhythm? Better inhibitory control is linked with more consistent drumming and enhanced neural tracking of the musical beat in adult percussionists and nonpercussionists. *Journal of Cognitive Neuroscience*, 30(1), 14–24.

Sloboda, J.A. (1985). *The Musical Mind: The Cognitive Psychology of Music*. Oxford: Clarendon Press.

Smith, A., Taylor, E., Warner Rogers, J., Newman, S. & Rubia, K. (2002). Evidence for a pure time perception deficit in children with ADHD. *Journal of Child Psychology and Psychiatry*, 43(4), 529–542.

Smith, D.J., Stepp, C., Guenther, F.H. & Kearney, E. (2020). Contributions of auditory and somatosensory feedback to vocal motor control. *Journal of Speech, Language, and Hearing Research*, 63(7), 2039–2053.

Solomon, N.P. & Charron, S. (1998). Speech breathing in able-bodied children and children with cerebral palsy: A review of the literature and implications for clinical intervention. *American Journal of Speech-Language Pathology*, 7(2), 61–78.

Sousa, D.A. (2016). *How the Brain Learns*. Newbury Park, CA: Corwin Press.

Soyucen, E. & Esen, F. (2010). Benign joint hypermobility syndrome: A cause of childhood asthma? *Medical Hypotheses*, 74(5), 823–824.

Sperdin, H.F. & Schaer, M. (2016). Aberrant development of speech processing in young children with autism: New insights from neuroimaging biomarkers. *Frontiers in Neuroscience*, 10, 393.

Srinivasan, S.M., Kaur, M., Park, I.K., Gifford, T.D., Marsh, K.L. & Bhat, A.N. (2015). The effects of rhythm and robotic interventions on the imitation/praxis, interpersonal synchrony, and motor performance of children with autism spectrum disorder (ASD): A pilot randomized controlled trial. *Autism Research and Treatment*, 2015, 736516. doi: 10.1155/2015/736516.

Stackhouse, J. & Wells, B. (1997). *Children's Speech and Literacy Difficulties: A Psycholinguistic Framework*. London: Whurr.

Stahl, B., Henseler, I., Turner, R., Geyer, S. & Kotz, S.A. (2013). How to engage the right brain hemisphere in aphasics without even singing: Evidence for two paths of speech recovery. *Frontiers in Human Neuroscience*, 7, 35.

Stamou, A., Bonneville Roussy, A., Ockelford, A. & Terzi, L. (2019). The effectiveness of a music and dance program on the task engagement and inclusion of young pupils on the autism spectrum. *Music & Science*, (2), 1–12. https://doi.org/10.1177/2059204319881852.

Stelmachowicz, P.G., Pittman, A.L., Hoover, B.M. & Lewis, D.E. (2004). Novel-word learning in children with normal hearing and hearing loss. *Ear and Hearing*, 25(1), 47–56.

Stephenson, J. (2006). Music therapy and the education of students with severe disabilities. *Education and Training in Developmental Disabilities*, 290–299.

Stepp, C.E., Lester-Smith, R.A., Abur, D., Daliri, A., Pieter Noordzij, J. & Lupiani, A.A. (2017). Evidence for auditory-motor impairment in individuals with hyperfunctional voice disorders. *Journal of Speech, Language, and Hearing Research*, 60(6), 1545–1550.

Stojanovik, V. (2011). Prosodic deficits in children with Down syndrome. *Journal of Neurolinguistics*, 24(2), 145–155.

Stormont, B. & Shepard, C. (2004). *Jabulani!: Ideas for Making Music (Education Series)*. Stroud: Hawthorn Press.

Stratford, B. & Ching, E.Y.Y. (1989). Responses to music and movement in the development of children with Down's syndrome. *Journal of Intellectual Disability Research*, 33(1), 13–24.

Stuart, N. (2016) *Way to Play Handbook.* Petone, Lower Hutt: Autism NZ.

Suppanen, E., Huotilainen, M. & Ylinen, S. (2019). Rhythmic structure facilitates learning from auditory input in newborn infants. *Infant Behavior and Development*, 57, 101346.

Swaminathan, S. & Schellenberg, E.G. (2020). Musical ability, music training, and language ability in childhood. *Journal of Experimental Psychology: Learning, Memory, and Cognition*, 46(12), 2340.

Szczygieł, E., Blaut, J., Zielonka-Pycka, K., Tomaszewski, K. *et al.* (2018). The impact of deep muscle training on the quality of posture and breathing. *Journal of Motor Behavior*, 50(2), 219–227.

Tannock, R. (2018). ADHD and Communication Disorders. In T. Banaschewski, D. Coghill & A. Zuddas (eds), *Oxford Textbook of Attention Deficit Hyperactivity Disorder*, pp.261–272. Oxford: Oxford University Press.

Taylor, J.E.T. & Witt, J.K. (2015). Listening to music primes space: Pianists, but not novices, simulate heard actions. *Psychological Research*, 79(2), 175–182.

Thaut, M.H. (2005). Neurologic Music Therapy Techniques and Definitions. In M. Thaut, *Rhythm, Music and the Brain: Scientific Foundations and Clinical Applications.* New York, NY: Routledge.

Thoen, A., Alaerts, K., Steyaert, J. & Van Damme, T. (2021). Respiratory sinus arrhythmia biofeedback to reduce physiological stress in adolescents with autism spectrum disorder. In *International Conference of Physiotherapy in Psychiatry and Mental Health,* 2021, Location: Helsinki, Finland.

Titze, I.R. & Martin, D.W. (1994). *Principles of Voice Production.* Hoboken, NJ: Prentice Hall.

Torppa, R. & Huotilainen, M. (2019). Why and how music can be used to rehabilitate and develop speech and language skills in hearing-impaired children. *Hearing Research*, 380, 108–122.

Torres, E.B. & Donnellan, A.M. (eds) (2015). *Autism: The Movement Perspective.* Lausanne, Switzerland: Frontiers Media SA.

Trainor, L.J., Clark, E.D., Huntley, A. & Adams, B.A. (1997). The acoustic basis of preferences for infant-directed singing. *Infant Behavior and Development*, 20(3), 383–396.

Trehub, S.E. & Hannon, E.E. (2009). Conventional rhythms enhance infants' and adults' perception of musical patterns. *Cortex*, 45(1), 110–118.

Trevarthen, C. (1999). Musicality and the intrinsic motive pulse: Evidence from human psychobiology and infant communication. *Musicae Scientiae*, 3(1_ suppl), 155–215.

Trevarthen, C. (2008). The musical art of infant conversation: Narrating in the time of sympathetic experience, without rational interpretation, before words. *Musicae Scientiae*, 12(1_suppl), 15–46.

Trevarthen, C. (2009). The functions of emotion in infancy. *The Healing Power of Emotion*, 55–85.

Trevarthen, C. & Delafield-Butt, J.T. (2013). Autism as a developmental disorder in intentional movement and affective engagement. *Frontiers in Integrative Neuroscience*, 7, 49.

Turnbull, F. (2018). *Learning with Music: Games and Activities for the Early Years*. Abingdon, Oxfordshire: Routledge.

Unwin, L.M., Bruz, I., Maybery, M.T., Reynolds, V. *et al.* (2017). Acoustic properties of cries in 12-month old infants at high-risk of autism spectrum disorder. *Journal of Autism and Developmental Disorders*, 47(7), 2108–2119.

Vaiouli, P. & Andreou, G. (2018). Communication and language development of young children with autism: A review of research in music. *Communication Disorders Quarterly*, 39(2), 323–329.

van Leeuwen, T.M., Neufeld, J., Hughes, J. & Ward, J. (2020). Synaesthesia and autism: Different developmental outcomes from overlapping mechanisms? *Cognitive Neuropsychology*, 37(7–8), 433–449.

Vance, S. (2017). *Music as the Architect for Speech and Language: A Systematic Review*. https://scholarworks.gvsu.edu/cgi/viewcontent.cgi?article=1662&context=honorsprojects.

Vaquero, L., Rousseau, P.N., Vozian, D., Klein, D. & Penhune, V. (2020). What you learn & when you learn it: Impact of early bilingual & music experience on the structural characteristics of auditory-motor pathways. *NeuroImage*, 213, 116689.

Vilhauer, R.P. (2017). Characteristics of inner reading voices. *Scandinavian Journal of Psychology*, 58(4), 269–274.

Vygotsky, L.S. (1978). *Mind in Society: The Development of Higher Psychological Processes*. Cambridge, MA: Harvard University Press.

Wan, C.Y. & Schlaug, G. (2013). Brain Plasticity Induced by Musical Training. In D. Deutsch (ed.), *The Psychology of Music*, pp.565–581. New York, NY: Academic Press.

Wan, C.Y., Bazen, L., Baars, R., Libenson, A. *et al.* (2011). Auditory-motor mapping training as an intervention to facilitate speech output in non-verbal children with autism: A proof of concept study. *PloS One*, 6(9), e25505.

Wan, C., Ruber, T., Hohmann, A. & Schlaug, G. (2010). The therapeutic effects of singing in neurological disorders. *Music Perception*, 27(4), 287–296.

Wang, X., Wang, S., Fan, Y., Huang, D. & Zhang, Y. (2017). Speech-specific categorical perception deficit in autism: An event-related potential study of lexical tone processing in Mandarin-speaking children. *Scientific Reports*, 7(1), 1–12.

Ward, J. (2021). Synaesthesia as a model system for understanding variation in the human mind and brain. *Cognitive Neuropsychology*, 1–20.

Welch, G.F. (1985). Variability of practice and knowledge of results as factors in learning to sing in tune. *Bulletin of the Council for Research in Music Education*, 238–247.

Welch, G.F. (1998). Early childhood musical development. *Research Studies in Music Education*, 11(1), 27–41. http://doi.org/10.1177/1321103X9801100104.

Welch, G.F. (2005). Singing as communication. *Musical Communication*, 1, 239–259.

Welch, G.F. (2009). Evidence of the development of vocal pitch matching ability in children 1. *Japanese Journal of Music Education Research*, 21, 1–13.

Welch, G.F. (2015). Singing and Vocal Development. In G. McPherson (ed.), *The Child as Musician: A Handbook of Musical Development*. Oxford: Oxford University Press.

Welch, G.F., Himonides, E., Saunders, J., Papageorgi, I. & Sarazin, M. (2014). Singing and social inclusion. *Frontiers in Psychology*, 5, 803.

Welch, G.F., Himonides, E., Saunders, J., Papageorgi, I. *et al.* (2008). The national singing programme for primary schools in England: An initial baseline study overview, February 2008. Institute of Education, University of London.

Welch, G.F., Howard, D.M. & Rush, C. (1989). Real-time visual feedback in the development of vocal pitch accuracy in singing. *Psychology of Music,* 17(2), 146–157.

Welsh, T.N., Elliott, D. & Simon, D.A. (2003). Cerebral specialization and verbal-motor integration in adults with and without Down syndrome. *Brain and Language,* 84(2), 152–169.

Wenhart, T., Bethlehem, R.A., Baron-Cohen, S. & Altenmueller, E. (2019). Autistic traits, resting-state connectivity, and absolute pitch in professional musicians: Shared and distinct neural features. *Molecular Autism,* 10(1), 1–18.

West, M.L. (1992). *Ancient Greek Music.* Oxford: Clarendon Press.

Whiteside, S.P., Inglis, A.L., Dyson, L., Roper, A. *et al.* (2012). Error reduction therapy in reducing struggle and grope behaviours in apraxia of speech. *Neuropsychological Rehabilitation,* 22(2), 267–294.

Willemin, T., Litchke, L.G., Liu, T., & Ekins, C. (2018). Social emotional effects of Drumtastic*: A dyadic within-group drumming pilot program for children with autism spectrum disorder. *International Journal of Special Education,* 33(1), 94–103.

Williams, D. (1996). *Autism – An Inside-Out Approach: An Innovative Look at the Mechanics of 'Autism' and Its Developmental Cousins.* London: Jessica Kingsley Publishers.

Williams, J. (2018). *Teaching Singing to Children and Young Adults* (second edition). Abingdon, Oxfordshire: Compton Publishing.

Williamson, V. (2014). *You Are the Music: How Music Reveals What It Means to Be Human.* London: Icon Books.

Wilson, M. & Cook, P.F. (2016). Rhythmic entrainment: Why humans want to, fireflies can't help it, pet birds try, and sea lions have to be bribed. *Psychonomic Bulletin & Review,* 23(6), 1647–1659.

Wisniewski, M.G., Mantell, J.T. & Pfordresher, P.Q. (2013). Transfer effects in the vocal imitation of speech and song. *Psychomusicology: Music, Mind, and Brain,* 23(2), 82.

Wong, B., Brebner, C., McCormack, P. & Butcher, A. (2015). Word production inconsistency of Singaporean-English-speaking adolescents with Down Syndrome. *International Journal of Language & Communication Disorders,* 50(5), 629–645.

Wood, L., Ivery, P., Donovan, R. & Lambin, E. (2013). 'To the beat of a different drum': Improving the social and mental wellbeing of at-risk young people through drumming. *Journal of Public Mental Health,* 12(2), 70–79.

Wynn, C.J., Borrie, S.A. & Sellers, T.P. (2018). Speech rate entrainment in children and adults with and without autism spectrum disorder. *American Journal of Speech-Language Pathology,* 27(3), 965–974.

Yardımcı-Lokmanoğlu, B.N., Bingöl, H. & Mutlu, A. (2020). The forgotten sixth sense in cerebral palsy: Do we have enough evidence for proprioceptive treatment? *Disability and Rehabilitation,* 42(25), 3581–3590.

Zampini, L., Fasolo, M., Spinelli, M., Zanchi, P., Suttora, C. & Salerni, N. (2016). Prosodic skills in children with Down syndrome and in typically developing children. *International Journal of Language & Communication Disorders,* 51(1), 74–83.

Ziethe, A., Petermann, S., Hoppe, U., Greiner, N., Brüning, M., Bohr, C. & Döllinger, M. (2019). Control of fundamental frequency in dysphonic patients during phonation and speech. *Journal of Voice*, 33(6), 851–859.

Zoefel, B., Ten Oever, S. & Sack, A.T. (2018). The involvement of endogenous neural oscillations in the processing of rhythmic input: More than a regular repetition of evoked neural responses. *Frontiers in Neuroscience*, 12, 95.

Zoller, M.B. (1991). Use of music activities in speech-language therapy. *Language, Speech, and Hearing Services in Schools*, 22(1), 272–276.

Zuk, J., Benjamin, C., Kenyon, A. & Gaab, N. (2014). Behavioral and neural correlates of executive functioning in musicians and non-musicians. *PloS One*, 9(6), e99868.

Zylowska, L., Ackerman, D.L., Yang, M.H., Futrell, J.L. *et al.* (2008). Mindfulness meditation training in adults and adolescents with ADHD: A feasibility study. *Journal of Attention Disorders*, 11(6), 737–746.

Subject Index

Author Index